INTRODUCTION TO
FUNCTIONAL
HUMAN
ANATOMY

W. B. Saunders Company:

West Washington Square
Philadelphia, Pa. 19105

12 Dyott Street
London, WC1A 1DB

833 Oxford Street
Toronto 18, Ontario

© 1970 N.V. Uitgeversmaatschappij De Tijdstroom
   Lochem, The Netherlands.

Library of Congress catalog card number 73-76188.

ISBN 0-7216-7945-5

introduction to
FUNCTIONAL
HUMAN
ANATOMY
an atlas

JOHANNES P. SCHADÉ, M.D., PH.D.
Associate Director, Central Institute for Brain Research;
Lecturer in Neurophysiology, University of Utrecht; Director,
Medical Library Foundation, Utrecht, The Netherlands

W. B. Saunders Company/Philadelphia/London/Toronto

PREFACE

This book was first conceived some five years ago in response to an evident need for a concise introductory course for students interested in the structure and function of the human body.

In recent years the teaching of anatomy and physiology has undergone profound changes. Nowhere is the student exposed to the old style of detailed instruction. This presentation is based more on pictures than on words.

Introduction to Functional Human Anatomy gives a complete survey of human anatomy, with reference to the functional significance of the structures. The book has been extensively illustrated so that a wide range of students from various disciplines may readily "see" what they are reading.

JOHANNES P. SCHADÉ

CONTENTS

PLATES

ATLAS OF THE HUMAN BODY

The foundations of our present knowledge of human anatomy were laid as early as the 16th century and now form the basis of contemporary medicine.

Thorough familiarity with the structure and development of the body is indispensable for the science as well as for the practice of medicine.

Through the decades, human anatomy has developed from a static into a dynamic science. By describing the structure of the human body, we attempt to obtain a deeper insight into its functional role. Structure and function are inseparable.

Although the body must be regarded as an integral unit, it is necessary that organ systems forming parts of it be discussed separately. In doing so, we shall review the following order: the bones, joints, muscles, blood vessels, nerves, sense organs and internal organs.

In homage to the founder of modern anatomy, the Flemish physician Andreas Vesalius, each chapter is preceded by a plate from his famous textbook of anatomy, *De Humani Corporis Fabrica*. Vesalius lived from 1514 to 1564, and his textbook was published in 1543. Many of the plates in the original book were drawn by the Flemish artist Jan Stephaan van Kalcker, a disciple of Titian. Vesalius' book provoked so much professional resistance that he gave up his professorial chair and became court physician to Charles V and Philip II. His famous book has remained an inexhaustible source of information. A few years ago this monumental work was reproduced in facsimile.

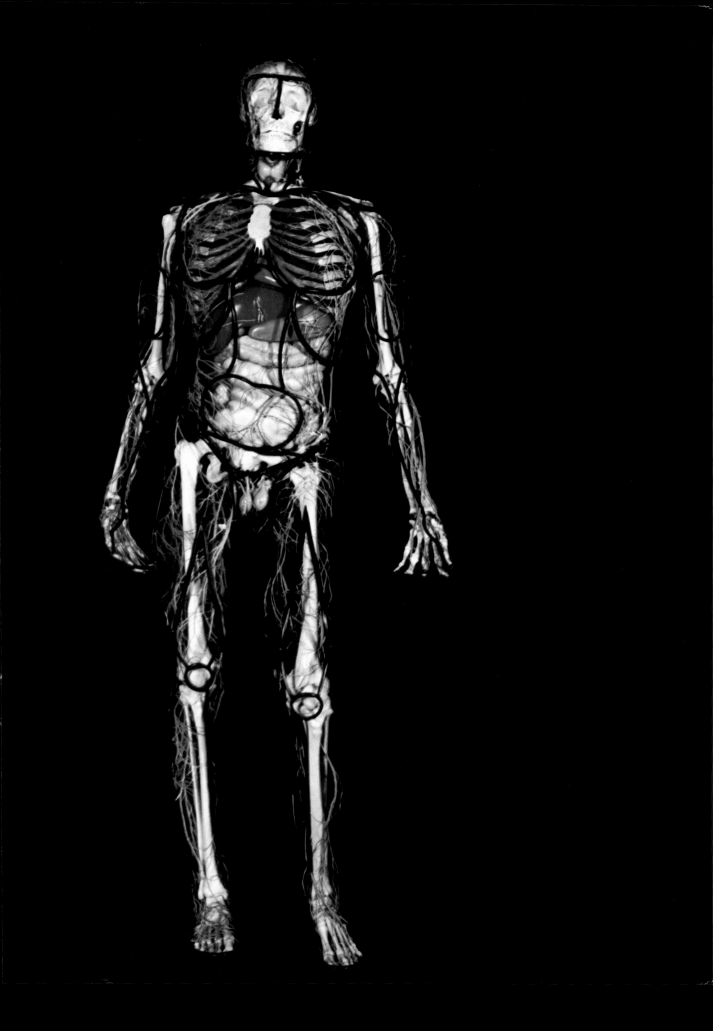

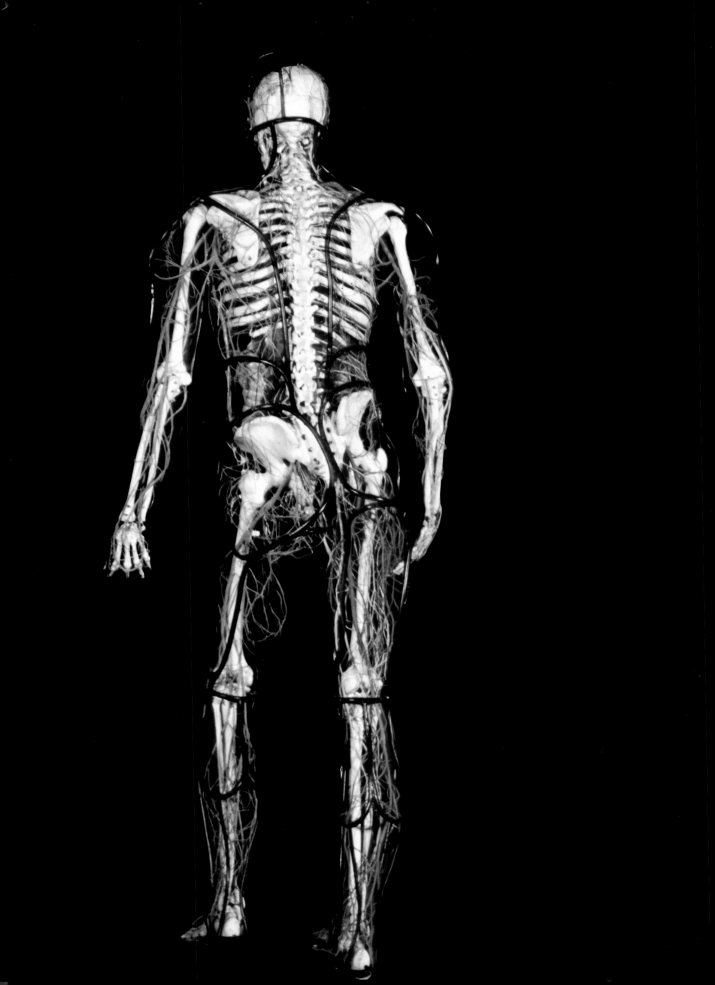

This atlas is divided into six sections, preceded by a brief discussion of the cells and tissues making up the various organs. Each section is illustrated by one or more folding color plates, the sequence of which makes a unique atlas of anatomy.

I   The skeleton and the joints (Plates A and B)
This is a survey of the microscopic structure of bone or osseous tissue, the ossification processes, the types and function of the joints, and the patterns of movement.

II   The muscular system (Plates C, D, E and F)
A discussion of the types of muscle tissue and the bio-mechanics of movement. A table enumerates more than 100 important muscles, showing their respective points of adhesion, innervation and function.

III   The heart and blood vessels (Plate G)
The circulatory system is composed of blood vessels of varying diameter, which, if placed end-to-end, would extend to a distance of about 200,000 kilometers. The main vessels are discussed, and the arteries are tabulated, showing their origin and the area they serve.

IV   The nervous system (Plates H and I)
The fine white strands visible to the naked eye under the skin and between the muscle are the nerves. Often they are formed of bundles of hundreds of nerve fibers. These nerves, with their sensory receptors, mediate between the individual and his environment, as does the brain, which is the seat of abstract thinking, memory and consciousness. The peripheral and central nervous systems are schematically illustrated.

V   The sense organs (Plate J)
These organs maintain contact with the external surroundings. The morphologic aspects of these complex organs are discussed.

VI   The internal organs (Plate K)
The internal organs are located primarily in the thorax, the abdomen, and the pelvis. This chapter deals with the respiratory, digestive, reproductive and urinary systems.

THE CELL AS A BUILDING BLOCK

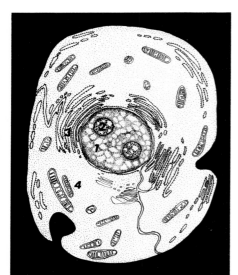

Schema of a cell

1. nucleus
2. nucleolus
3. endoplasmic reticulum
4. mitochondrion

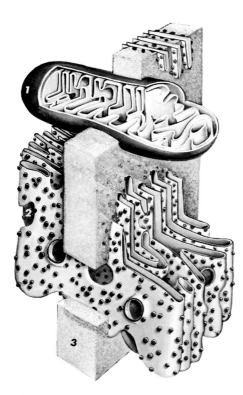

Electron micrograph of the three cell constituents

1. mitochondrion
2. endoplasmic reticulum
3. cytoplasm

The cell is the smallest unit possessing all the essential properties of a living organism, such as metabolism, reproduction, differentiation, regeneration, and excitability. *Metabolism* means the conversion of food into building blocks for the body. These building blocks are in turn broken down to provide energy for the cell. *Reproduction* in most multicellular organisms originates from a fertilized single cell that undergoes division a great many times to form a complete organism. This process is always coupled with growth. *Differentiation* is a process of cellular transformation resulting in the formation of specialized cell types. *Regeneration* is cellular restoration or repair. *Excitability* means the ability to respond to an adequate stimulus with a certain reaction. These life functions of the cell occur on a microscopic and submicroscopic level.

With the aid of the light microscope and the electron microscope, minute structural details of tissues and organs can be revealed. Although cells may have a wide variety of forms, depending on their specific function, all cells have the following components:

1. An outer cell membrane
2. Cytoplasm, i.e., the contents of the cell excluding the nucleus
3. A cell nucleus, more or less spherical, containing chromatin and a nucleolus
4. Organelles, i.e., cytoplasmic structures to which the diverse functions are attributed.

The cell membrane consists of a very thin layer of regularly arranged molecules of fat and proteins. The membrane is selectively permeable to certain substances. The nucleus is the carrier of genetic properties and, during the life of the cell, it plays a leading role that is indispensable to cellular activity. For this purpose, the nucleus contains a high concentration of nucleic acid (deoxyribonucleic acid, DNA) which stores all hereditary information or characteristics. The nucleolus residing in the nucleus is composed of ribonucleic acid (RNA). The cytoplasm also contains RNA. Together these two nucleic acids control cellular functions and are responsible for the production of proteins in the cell.

Of the many organelles in the cytoplasm, the most important are the mitochondria, the unbound RNA, the endoplasmic reticulum, and the Golgi apparatus. The mitochondria are round or elongate structures consisting of a complex system of double membranes to which enzymes are bound. Their main task is to supply energy for the cell's metabolism. Unbound RNA synthesizes proteins used within the cell. The endoplasmic reticulum (RNA bound to membranes) is a maze of concentric cavities wherein synthesized proteins are transported to the Golgi apparatus and prepared for discharge from the cell, as is the case in digestive enzyme producing cells (e.g., pancreatic exocrine gland cells).

From a single fertilized egg cell, the tissues, organs and, finally, the whole organism develop by cell division and differentiation. When a cell multiplies, daughter cells identical to the mother cell arise. Genetic characteristics are stored in the nucleus in the form of chromatin (DNA). During cell division, the chromatin is arranged in a ribbon shape, while the nuclear membrane disappears. The ribbon is then divided into a number of short strands, the chromosomes. The number of chromosomes is characteristic for each plant or animal. Man possesses 23 pairs of chromosomes, 22 of which are identical pairs; the other two are sex chromosomes. In the female, this pair consists of two identical chromosomes (XX); in the male, the two chromosomes are not identical (XY).

Several stages can be distinguished in cell division. The second of these, called metaphase, is characterized by a lengthwise splitting of the chromosomes. In the third stage, anaphase, the two halves of the split chromosomes move to opposite sides of the cell, where they aggregate to form new nuclei. At the end of this stage the entire cell divides and the process terminates with the disappearance of the chromosomes and the appearance of the nuclear membrane and two complete cells. This is called telophase. In this manner, the division of the mother cell results in two daughter cells.

From these first cells, complete organisms can develop. In a later stage, the ability to divide may be lost, and gradually cell differentiation comes to the fore. Groups of cells begin to specialize for the performance of certain functions; tissue formation begins. Tissues are groups of cells that have a common origin and function.

The development of sex cells is slightly different: in the fusion of a male sperm and female egg a cell is formed which contains the somatic number (twice the germ cell number) of chromosomes. The paired chromosomes of immature sex cells are divided, so that each daughter nucleus possesses only half the number of chromosomes of the mother nucleus. This is called the haploid number, in contrast to the diploid number of chromosomes that other cells contain. This process is called reduction. These cells become the sperm cells (spermatocytes) in the male and the egg cells (oocytes) in the female. During fertilization, a spermatocyte and an oocyte fuse, so that a new cell containing the diploid number of chromosomes forms.

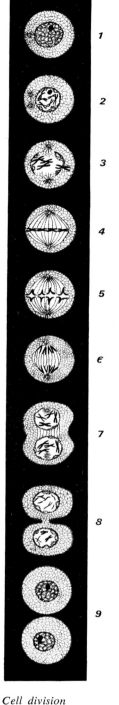

Cell division

1. mother cell
2. interphase
3. prometaphase
4. and 5. metaphase
6. and 7. anaphase
8. telophase
9. daughter cells

Male (1) and female (2) sex chromosomes

EPITHELIAL TISSUE

1

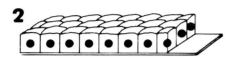

2

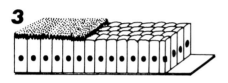

3

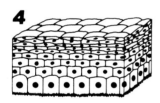

4

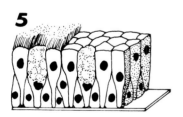

5

The body is composed of four kinds of primary tissues: epithelial, connective, muscle, and nerve.

The epithelium that covers the surface or lines a cavity of the body consists of one more layers of adjoining cells. Often, strands of cells grow from the epithelium into deeper lying layers and differentiate to form glands. Some sensory receptors are a specialized form of epithelium.

Epithelial cells are cells with diverse functions. Thus, the epidermis of the skin consists of a multilayered epithelium that is resistant to harmful external factors. Cell division occurs only in the lowest layers. The gastrointestinal epithelium has a completely different function. Here, the epithelium forms a single layer of cylindrical cells lying close together like multiangular blocks. It is the responsibility of these cells to absorb and transport digested foods from the intestinal lumen. The external surface of the cells is covered with a thin layer of mucus, which is produced by another cell type (goblet cells) and which has a protective role.

The epithelial cells of the respiratory organs are also well adapted for their specific function. There is a single layer of elongated cells covered with a mucous coat. The surface of these cells is ciliated to expel inhaled dust particles toward the mouth and nose. The cilia are anchored near the surface of the cell; their movement is in waves, with swift strokes in the direction of the nose and mouth and slow strokes in the opposite direction. In the lobules, the epithelial cells are extremely thin, permitting easy exchange of oxygen and carbon dioxide with the blood located in the capillaries.

Where the epithelial cells are specialized as in glands, they have a characteristic structure. Frequently the cells secrete their products directly on an external surface of the body. These glands are called exocrine glands. In certain parts of the body, some glands produce hormones which are secreted internally into the blood, to be carried to other organs. These are called endocrine glands. In contrast to the exocrine glands, they possess no ducts and are called ductless glands.

Epithelial tissues

1. single epithelial layer
2. cuboidal epithelial layer
3. cylindrical epithelium
4. multilayered epithelium
5. ciliated epithelium

CONNECTIVE TISSUE

This tissue is so named because it constitutes the connective and supporting element of the body. Connective tissue has various forms, such as fibrous bands, fat, blood, and bone.

These tissues are all derived from a common basic plan still recognizable in a number of characteristics shared by all. The tissues consist of cells separated by an intermediary substance or medium which has differentiated into both amorphous and formed elements, the former being the *matrix* and the latter the *fibers*. The matrix is a jelly-like mass containing a variable number of fibers. Young cartilage is composed of a large number of cells surrounded by a firm matrix which contains a small number of fibers.

Mature tissue is differentiated in many ways. For example, blood consists of a liquid matrix containing cells and fibers in a solubilized form. The development of supporting tissue, such as cartilage and bone, results in cells being enclosed in a matrix which has a firm or hard composition.

Fibers can be divided into three types: elastic, reticular, and collagenous. For example, elastic fibers are found in some cartilage, reticular fibers in fat tissue, and collagenous fibers in bone and cartilage.

During the formation of blood from immature connective tissue the cells and pupporting tissue undergo great changes. At a certain time during fetal life, the connective tussue cells in some parts of the embryo flatten and aggregate to form membranous ducts. This is the initial layout for the blood vessels of the circulatory system. The cells contained inside these primitive vessels become rounded and the medium becomes liquid, forming the earliest blood. In a later stage, the vessels become joined in a continuous system and the heart begins to develop. When this has been achieved and the heart begins to pump, the blood inside the vessels begins to move, initiating blood circulation. The liquid matrix of the blood can also become solidified; during clotting, theads called fibrin are formed.

Loose connective tissue is found primarily under the skin, between organs and their parts. It consists of few cells and variable amounts of elastic, reticular, and collagenous fibers. Fat tissue, which contains large numbers of fat cells, is also a loose connective tissue. The nucleus of the fat cell is pushed to one side and the cell is filled with a round ball of fat. The fat cells function partly as a storage depot (to be drawn on when food intake is insufficient) and partly as protection (temperature loss) and tissue support.

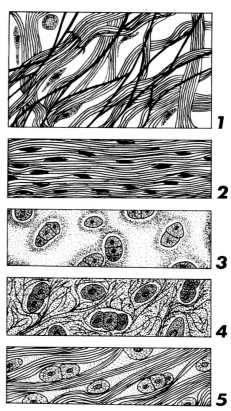

Connective tissue

1. elastic and collagenous fibers of the connective tissue
2. connective tissue with many collagenous
3. hyaline cartilage
4. elastic cartilage
5. fibrous cartilage

1

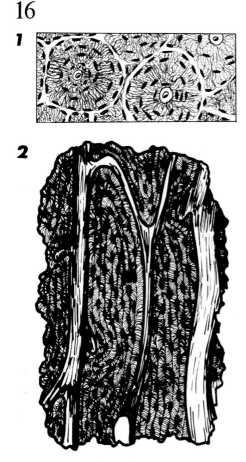

2

Organization of bone tissue

1. cross section
2. longitudinal section

Precipitation of certain substances into the matrix of fibrous connective tissue allows cartilage to be formed through solidification of the original tissues. Cartilage consists of a matrix containing small groups of cells. The matrix is a mesh of fibers imbedded in an amorphous medium.

The division of cartilage cells (chondrocytes) results in daughter cells, which also produce matrix, contributing to the growth of cartilage. This phenomenon is called internal or interstitial growth, and is represented by clusters of chondrocytes, called family groups. There are no blood vessels in cartilage, so that diffusion of nutrients plays an essential role in its metabolism.

According to microscopic structure, several types of cartilage can be distinguished:

a. Hyaline cartilage is found in joints and contains few fibers. It has a smooth, glassy appearance and its consistency is comparable to hard rubber. Its elasticity allows it to distribute pressure evenly over the ends of the bones in a joint.
b. Fibrocartilage is primarily found in the discs between the spinal vertebrae. It is both pliable and solid in form.
c. Elastic cartilage contains a large number of elastic fibers and can be easily bent, but will recover its original shape afterward. A typical example is the cartilage of the auricle of the ear.

Cartilage is found in many other structures in the body—the tip and septum of the nose, the rings of the trachea and bronchi and of the larynx, and the anterior portion of the ribs.

When calcium salts accumulate in the matrix of connective tissue, it becomes brittle and hard. This is how bone tissue is formed. It can arise in two ways: directly from connective tissue or indirectly via an intermediate phase of cartilage. Bones contain many blood vessels, which have, for the most part, a longitudinal course; they are surrounded by concentric layers of calcium salts. Between these layers are bone cells that maintain contact with each other by means of tiny cell processes. Also, the original connective tissue can still be seen; microscopically, the fibers can be detected in the calcium as tiny dots. Bone is by no means dead matter, as its tissue is subjected to constant building up and breaking down processes. Calcium salts can be withdrawn from bone not only under pathologic conditions (metabolic diseases, bone diseases) but also under normal circumstances (pregnancy). Loss of calcium is detrimental to the integrity of the bone. Moreover, bone normally serves also as a calcium depot for the body.

Muscle cells are distinguished by their capacity to contract. Of the three types of muscle — smooth, cardiac and skeletal — each has its specific structure and function.

Smooth muscle is composed of small spindle-shaped cells with a long cylindrical nucleus. The cells contain thin, contractile threads (myofilaments) that can be seen only under the electron microscope. Smooth muscle is found in layers, as, for example, in the walls of the arteries and the intestines.

The wall of the heart contains striated muscle. These large cells are highly branched. The striations are due to the presence of fibrils (myofibrils) that are known to be responsible for contractility. In certain areas, specialized cardiac muscle fibers called Purkinje fibers are seen; these contract poorly but conduct excitatory stimuli.

The cross-striated, skeletal muscle fibers are giant cylindrical cells. They are filled with bundles of parallel myofibrils composed primarily of contractile proteins, and have numerous nuclei which lie near the external membrane of the muscle fiber. Each muscle fiber is a long, cylindrical multinucleate cell reaching a length of 10 to 12 cm, with a diameter of 10 to 100 microns. A skeletal muscle consists of many such fibers or cells closely packed and lying parallel to each other. These cells are bound together with connective tussue containing many capillary blood vessels and a large number of nerve fibers.

The building blocks of the nervous system are the neurons. In form and function, they are cells specialized to receive and transmit stimuli. For this function, the neuron is equipped with a large number of richly branched shoots called dendrites, whose role is to receive impulses, and with an axon that conveys these impulses to other cells. The specific function of the nerve cell takes place along its external limiting membrane. In most cases, the axon is wrapped in a myelin sheath, which is specialized for insulating the axon. Contact between nerve cells is maintained by the synapses, i.e., the junction of axon endings with dendrite and nerve cell bodies.

Nerve tissue contains a second type of cell, the neuroglial cell. Its functions are to transport substances into the nervous system, to produce myelin sheaths, and to phagocytize cellular debris and other unwanted substances.

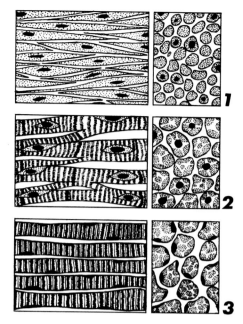

Muscle tissue

1. smooth muscle
2. cardiac muscle
3. skeletal muscle
left: longitudinal section
right: cross section

Schematic diagram of a nerve cell and its connection with a cross-striated muscle fiber

a. cell body
b. nucleus and nucleolus
c. dendrite
d. axonal end of a cell making synaptic contact
e. axon
f. myelin sheath
g. node of Ranvier
h. myoneural synapse
i. cross-striated muscle
j. neuroplasm of a cell body with mitochondria and the endoplasmic reticulum.

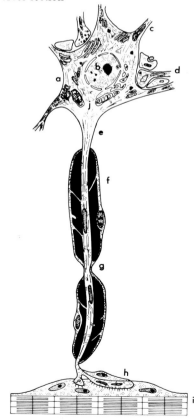

MICROGRAPHS OF CELLS AND TISSUES

The structure of cells and tissues can be studied under the microscope, by making thin slices (sections) of the material. The tissue is then stained with a dye or dyes specific for one or more of the cell components.

1. Micrograph of an onion root tip, showing several phases of cell division. In such a preparation, the various phases can be shown side by side.

2. Micrograph of a single-layer epithelium, such as that lining the pulmonary lobules.

3. Micrograph of intestinal epithelium, serving as an example for a single-layer cylindrical epithelium. The blue-stained material is mucus produced by goblet cells.

4. Micrograph of loose connective tissue. The cells lie within the maze of the connective tissue.

5. Micrograph of bone tissue. The concentric pattern of the osteons is clearly visible.

1

2

3

4

5

6

9

7

10

8

11

6. Micrograph of cross-striated muscle tissue stained with iron hematoxylin to show the striation pattern.

7. Micrograph of smooth muscle tissue, as found in the uterus.

8. The following micrographs show nerve tissues. Using various staining techniques, the many components of the nervous system can be pointed out. The cell body of a neuron (Bodian stain), revealing the many dendrites of a nerve cell.

9. Nerve cell from the spinal cord stained with cresyl violet. The nucleic acids in the cytoplasm have a marked affinity for this stain. The nucleus and the nucleolus can also be clearly discerned.

10. A group of nerve cells localized in the cerebral cortex, stained by the *Golgi-Cox* method. This method reveals only a small percentage of the nerve cells, but is most suitable for examination of the numerous shoots and dendrites of the nerve cells, together with their interconnections.

11. High magnification of a nerve cell, stained according to Golgi-Cox. The micrograph demonstrates the wealth of dendrites and dendritic branches sprouting from a nerve cell.

SKELETON AND JOINTS

The skeleton is the hard framework that supports the soft parts of the body. It comprises more than 200 bones, almost all of which are connected by means of the joints; together with the muscles, they form the apparatus of movement. The more vulnerable organs, such as the brain and spinal cord, are completely encased in bone, and the heart and lungs are protected by a cage formed by the ribs.

The many parts of the skeleton form a system of levers, by means of which the muscles can perform their work. Yet, the function of the skeleton is not merely static: it is also the site where blood cells are made, and, in addition, it serves as a depot for inorganic substances. Bone is thus not inert matter; it is continuously renewed through the breaking down of old constituents and the building of new ones.

Full growth of the skeleton continues for several decades until, at around the thirtieth year of age, its development is completed.

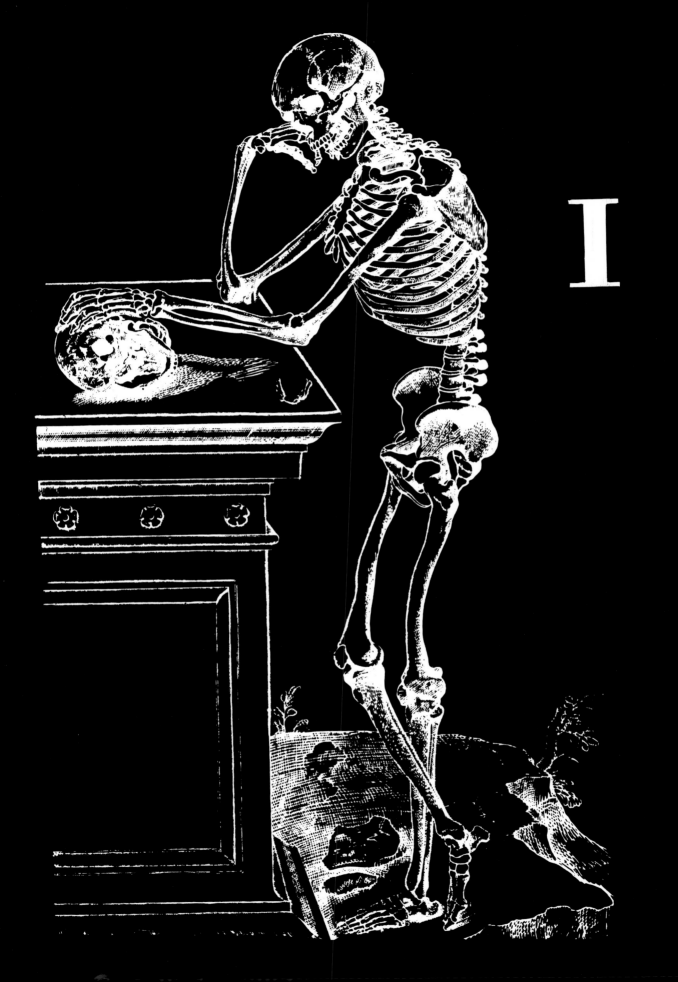

I

In studying and discussing the structure of the human body, a precise language is required. Specific terms for the exact notation of bodily sites are also essential to avoid an avalanche of incoherent data. "In front", "behind", "above", and "under" are place determinations that lose their significance when the position is altered, e.g., from standing to supine position. Thus, the definition of directions and planes in the body provides more accurate descriptions.

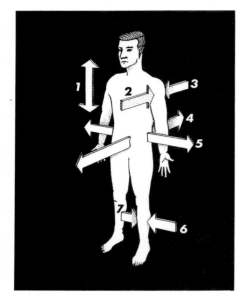

Planes

1. median plane
2. sagittal plane
3. frontal plane
4. transverse plane

Planes

Median: lying in the middle
> median plane: the plane dividing the body into two symmetrical parts
> medial: nearer the median plane
> medianly: lying or running in the direction of the median plane

Sagittal (sagitta = arrow): from front to rear (in the direction of an arrow shot)
> sagittal plane: any plane in the body in sagittal direction. Sagittal planes are parallel to the median plane.

Frontal: (frons = forehead): with respect to or belonging to the foremost part or the front side of the body or an organ (also with respect to the forehead)
> frontal plane: plane running the length of the body at right angles to the median plane

Transverse (transversalis, transversus, diagonal, across)
> transverse plane: across the width of the body. Median, frontal and transverse planes are at right angles to each other.

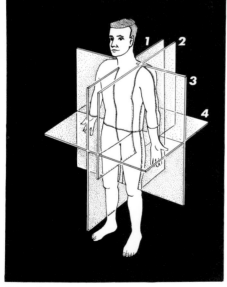

Directions

1. cranial and caudal
2. ventral and volar
3. dorsal
4. medial
5. transverse
6. lateral
7. medial

Directions

Cranial (cranium = skull): toward the skull, with respect to the skull

Caudal (cauda = tail): toward the tail or with respect to the tail (underside)

Ventral (venter = belly, stomach): with respect to the front part (belly) of the body (also anterior)

Dorsal (dorsum = back): with respect to the hind part (back) of the body (also posterior)

Volar (vola = palm of the hand): pertaining to the palm of the hand

Plantar (planta = sole of the foot): pertaining to the sole of the foot, toward the sole

P L A T E A
SKELETON
(front view)

Plaat Nr. 2000/1
Deutsches Hygiene-Museum,
Dresden

25 – 30

PLATE A
SKELETON
(front view)

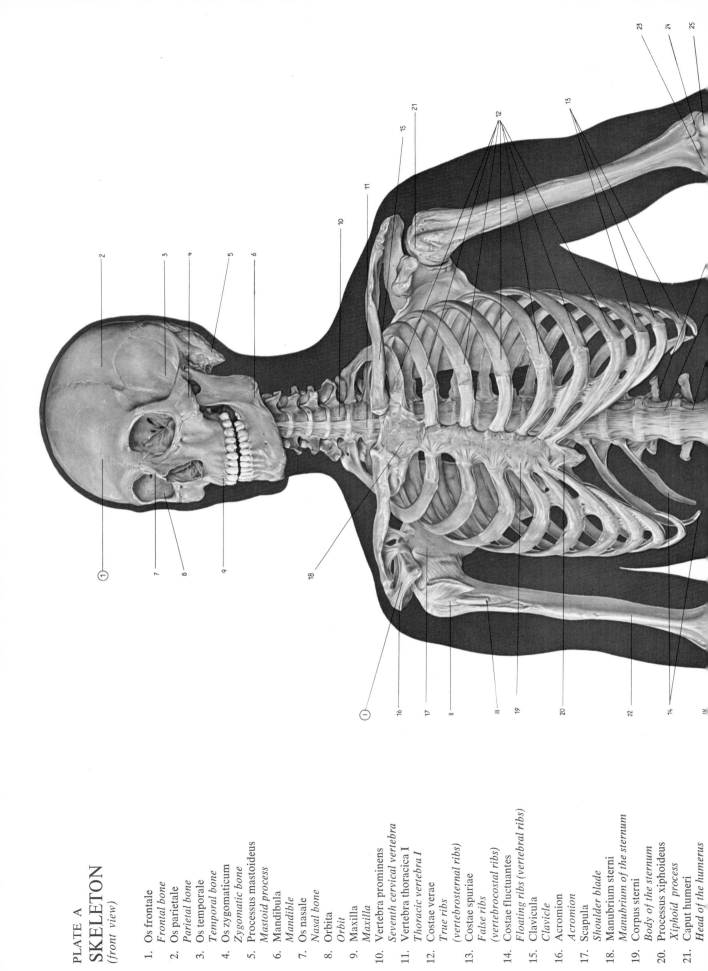

1. Os frontale
    Frontal bone
2. Os parietale
    Parietal bone
3. Os temporale
    Temporal bone
4. Os zygomaticum
    Zygomatic bone
5. Processus mastoideus
    Mastoid process
6. Mandibula
    Mandible
7. Os nasale
    Nasal bone
8. Orbita
    Orbit
9. Maxilla
    Maxilla
10. Vertebra prominens
    Seventh cervical vertebra
11. Vertebra thoracica I
    Thoracic vertebra I
12. Costae verae
    True ribs
    (vertebrosternal ribs)
13. Costae spuriae
    False ribs
    (vertebrocostal ribs)
14. Costae fluctuantes
    Floating ribs (vertebral ribs)
15. Clavicula
    Clavicle
16. Acromion
    Acromion
17. Scapula
    Shoulder blade
18. Manubrium sterni
    Manubrium of the sternum
19. Corpus sterni
    Body of the sternum
20. Processus xiphoideus
    Xiphoid process
21. Caput humeri
    Head of the humerus

THE SKELETON

The locomotor apparatus provides for the posture and movement of the body. It is made up of bones, joints, and muscles.

This chapter deals with *osteology,* the science of bones, and *syndesmology,* the science of connections among the bones. The skeleton consists of 212 bones in addition to 12 to 20 *sesamoid bones* (tiny bits of bone located within a number of tendons of the hand and foot muscles) and the teeth. The bones can be differentiated into *long bones,* such as the femur or thigh bone and the bones of legs and arms, and *flat bones,* such as the sternum or breast bone, the scapula or shoulder blade, and most cranial bones. In an adult, the total weight of the skeleton is about 10 kg, the femur being the heaviest single bone (1 kg). It is very strong, e.g., the femur can resist a pressure or pull of 1700 to 1800 kg. This is due to the construction of bone, which gives maximal strength and support with a minimum of weight.

Bone consists of cells and interstitial matter, the latter being composed of an organic fraction (ossein) in which numerous fibers are imbedded, and an inorganic fraction, consisting mainly of calcium and phosphorus. The density of bone is due to interstitial matter, while hardness results from calcium salts. The basic structure of the bone tissue is the *osteon,* a small canal surrounded by lamellae in which the fibers are arranged in a definite pattern. Located at the border of the lamellae are the bone cells, the *osteocytes.* When we look at a section of bone, we find a solid outer layer (substantia compacta) and a spongy inner layer (substantia spongiosa).

In compact bone, the osteons lie close to each other in a parallel arrangement, while in the spongy layer, they are spaced farther apart. Especially to be found in the long bones are remarkable *trabeculae,* or bony pillars, that are arranged to resist the pressure and pulling forces to which the bone is exposed. This arrangement is an excellent example of rational architectonic structure. The spongy part of many bones appears red, because their cavities contain a mass of red pigment found in developing red blood cells. In many long bones, the bone marrow appears yellow owing to the presence of numerous fat cells.

Numbers of Skeletal Bones

skull	25	pelvis	6
spinal column	34	legs	6
thorax	25	feet	52
shoulder girdle	4		
arms	6	Total	212
hands	54		

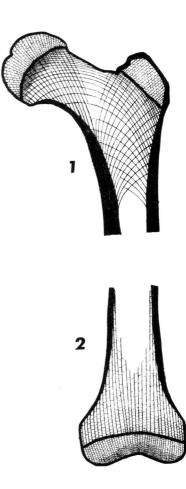

Section through the proximal (1) and distal (2) parts of the thigh bone, showing the trabecular organization

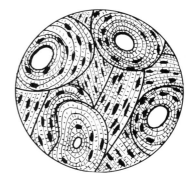

A foursome of osteons

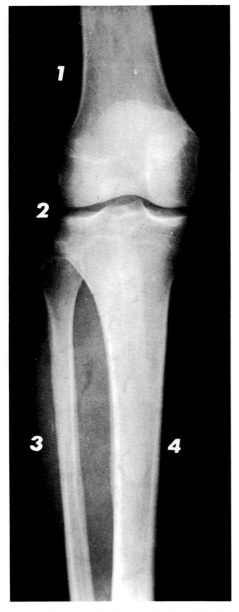

X-ray photograph of part of the right leg

1. femur
2. knee joint
3. fibula
4. tibia

Embryonal bone begins to form connective tissue at specific times in the fetus. Sometimes bone arises directly from connective tissue (intramembranous ossification), but more frequently via an intermediary cartilaginous stage (chondroid ossification).

An example of intramembranous ossification is seen in the cranial bones: new layers of bone are continuously deposited, until at last two conspicuous layers of bone are formed, with a spongy layer between; the latter contains many blood vessels.

The growth of the long bones is always preceded by a cartilaginous stage. Bone is first formed on the surface of the shaft (the *diaphysis);* thereafter blood vessels enter the shaft, and following this the marrow cavity is formed. At the extremities of the marrow cavity, a continuous process of chondroid ossification takes place. This zone is called the *metaphysis,* while the spongy extremities of the bone are named the *epiphyses.*

The growth process in the metaphysis has a twofold nature: on the side of the marrow cavity, cartilage is being transformed into bone, and at the epiphyses ample production of cartilage occurs. Much later — in most long bones only after birth — bone formation begins also at the epiphyses. Nevertheless, a cartilaginous disc, the epiphyseal plate, remains for several years between the metaphysis and the epiphyses; it has an important role in the growth in length of the long bone.

The growth period is most significant for the later life of any individual, for skeletal distortion and malformation can arise as a result of harmful influences. Deformities can result from loads disproportionate to skeletal resistance, due either to abnormally heavy loading or weakness of the skeleton.

During the lifetime of the individual, skeletal examination can be performed by x-rays. Of all body tissues, compact bones are the least permeable to these rays and will thus give a strong shadow on the film. A print made from the negative x-ray film will show the skeletal bones as white structures. Cartilage is not shown by x-rays but, from measurements of the distance between the bones at a joint, one can determine the place occupied by the cartilage. Muscle gives merely a vague shadow, the outlines of which can sometimes be seen.

Composition of Bone

water	50 %	copper	1.2%
fat	16 %	aluminum	0.5%
protein (collagen)	12.5%	manganese	0.2%
calcium	11 %	chlorine	0.2%
phosphorus	5 %	sodium	0.2%
lead	1.9%		

and minute quantities of silver, tin, etc.

THE TEETH

The upper and lower jaws are each equipped with a row of teeth, which are embedded in bone surrounded by a tight mucous membrane, the gingiva or gum. At about six months of age, the temporary or milk teeth appear, and their growth is completed by two years of age. There are 20 temporary teeth. From the sixth year, the temporary teeth are gradually pushed out to make place for the permanent teeth, of which the adult human has 32. Adult teeth have a variety of forms, corresponding to their respective functions. They are incisors, canines or eyeteeth, premolars or bicuspids, and molars or grinders. Number and disposition are schematically indicated by a formula using the initials of the Latin names of the teeth.

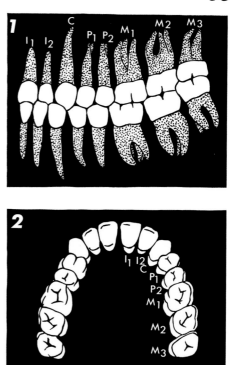

The formula for adult teeth is as follows:

$$\frac{I_1 \quad I_2 \quad C \quad P_1 \quad P_2 \quad M_1 \quad M_2 \quad M_3}{I_1 \quad I_2 \quad C \quad P_1 \quad P_2 \quad M_1 \quad M_2 \quad M_3}$$

that is, each half jaw has two incisors, one canine, two premolars, and three molars. Each tooth has a blood and nerve supply of its own.

Every tooth has a crown that stands out above the gum, a neck covered by the gum, and a root covered with a layer of cement, and is imbedded in a socket.

The tooth is mainly built up of dentin, a kind of hard bone, although the crown is covered with enamel, the composition of which is even harder than that of dentin. The dental periosteum (connective tissue) covers the roots and connects the tooth with the socket. Inside the tooth is a cavity containing the pulp, where the blood vessels and nerves are located. Through the canals of the root, the pulp cavity is connected with the surrounding tissue. The incisor has a chisel-shaped crown and a simple cylindrical root. The canine has a triangular point and a long, simple cylindrical root. The crown of the premolar has two cusps inside and outside; the root is split into two parts and is planted in the gum perpendicular to the row of teeth. The molar has a broad crown, with three to five cusps, and two or more roots. Of the twelve permanent molars the wisdom teeth are the smallest.

The incisors are used to cut through food, the canines for tearing it, and the molars for grinding it. Premolars have a function intermediate between canines and molars.

Teeth

1. side view
2. teeth of the lower jaw seen from above

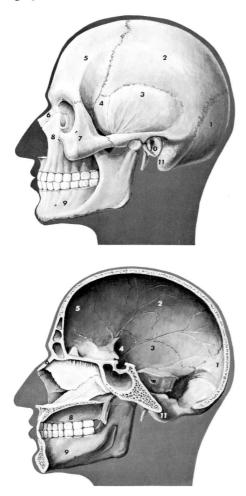

External and internal view of the skull

1. occipital bone
2. parietal bone
3. temporal bone
4. sphenoid bone
5. frontal bone
6. nasal bone
7. zygomatic bone
8. maxillary bone
9. mandibular bone
10. external auditory canal
11. mastoid process

THE SKULL

The bony structure of the head consists of two parts, the *cranium* and the *face*. The cranium is built of eight flat bones rigidly connected to each other. Most facial bones (upper jaw, hard palate, cheek bone) are also firmly grown together, but not the lower jaw, which moves in the jaw joint (temporomandibular joint).

THE SPINAL COLUMN

The vertebrae and the cartilaginous discs separating them provide firmness and mobility to the backbone or spinal column. The individual vertebrae are different in shape, the lower ones being bigger in order to cope with the heavier load they have to bear. The vertebrae do not form a straight pillar, as the spinal column is bent in a double S-shape. The seven cervical vertebrae and the five lumbar vertebrae present a forward curvature *(lordosis),* while the 12 thoracic vertebrae show a backward curvature *(kyphosis).* The lowest portion of the spinal column includes five fused vertebrae which make up the sacrum, and three or four fused vertebrae, which form the coccyx.

THE CHEST

A number of vital organs, such as the heart and the lungs, are well protected inside the chest. Its bony frame is made up of the breast bone or sternum and 12 pairs of ribs that are connected in the back with the dorsal vertebrae. Each rib can move by means of a hinge joint between two vertebral processes to which it is connected. The ribs are attached in front to the sternum by flexible pieces of cartilage.

THE ARM

The two bones on the right and the left side of the shoulder girdle, the shoulder blade (scapula) and the collar bone (clavicle), form an easy moving connection between the trunk and the upper extremity of the body. Thus, the role of the arms is clearly for grasping. The joints and bones of the forearm increase in number to facilitate differentiated grasping movements. The bones of the hand are divided into the carpals, metacarpals, and phalanges (finger bones).

THE LEG

The bones of the pelvic girdle reflect the function of the lower limbs. Both hip bones (consisting of the iliac bone, the hip bone, and the ischium (the seat bone), as well as the sacrum, are sturdy, massive, and built for stability. The ball (head) of the femur, the thigh bone, can revolve in the acetabulum or socket of the pelvis, which is composed of three fused bones.

The parts of the foot are the tarsus, the metatarsus, and the phalanges. The arched construction of the sole contributes greatly to the resilience of the gait. By coordinated movement of the many joints associated with the femur or thigh bone, the bones of the lower leg and feet, complicated actions such as walking or jumping become possible.

Joints, or articulations, occur where two bones or pieces of cartilage meet. The connection between them is maintained by ligaments and tendons of muscles.

Generally speaking, the functions of a joint are twofold:

a. to make movement possible, and
b. to form a solid tie between two pieces of bone.

The *fibrous junction* consists of connective tissue, such as the junction of cranial bones in children.

The *cartilaginous junction* is composed of cartilage; an example is the attachment of ribs to the sternum. In this case, movement is only moderately possible.

The *synovial junction* is the most familiar type of joint. The bone extremities facing each other are covered with a thin layer of smooth cartilage, with the synovial membrane and synovial fluid between them. The cartilage in the joint serves to reduce friction and to resist pressure. A closed sheath of fibrous tissue encapsulates the joint and is loose enough to permit movement in certain directions.

The ends of the opposite bones, covered with cartilage, are molded to fit together. Where they are not congruent, the ends of the bones are usually adapted to fit more perfectly by means of cartilaginous discs inserted between the two heads, such as the menisci of the knee joint. The cavity of the joint is a thin, fluid-filled slit. The synovial fluid, secreted by the synovial membrane of the capsule, not only lubricates the joint but also provides nutrients for the joint cartilage by diffusion.

The joint is usually supported by ligaments either within or outside the capsule; they assist in braking movements, and thus contribute to the stability of the joint. Mobility is greatest where the capsule is loose, e.g., in the shoulder joint, so that luxations (dislocations) can readily occur.

Two or more ends of bones can form a joint. Accordingly, we have a simple joint, formed by two bones, and a complex joint (articulatio composita), comprising several pieces of bone and cartilage.

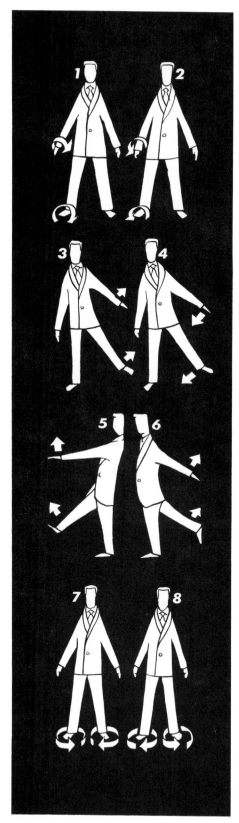

Movements

1. pronation of the arm and eversion of the foot
2. supination of the arm and inversion of the foot
3. abduction of arm and leg
4. adduction of arm and leg
5. anteflexion of arm and leg
6. retroflexion of arm and leg
7. endorotation
8. exorotation

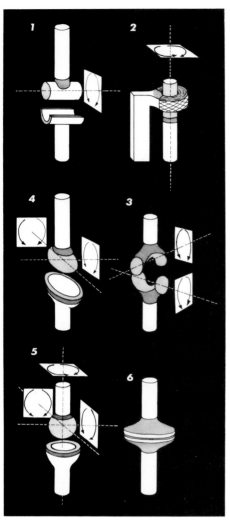

Schematic diagram of the various types of joints

1. hinge joint
2. rotating joint
3. saddle-shaped joint
4. egg-shaped joint
5. ball-shaped joint
6. immobile (fixed) joint

The broken lines indicate the axes of the joints

The mobility of a joint is, from the standpoint of its function, classified into three degrees of freedom — in other words, the freedom of moving the joints at right angles with respect to one another. For this reason, the notion of an axis of the joint has been introduced: in the illustration this is the broken line within the joint that is not involved in the movement, or actually the line about which the joint moves. We have joints with one, two, or three axes.

1. the hinge joint *(ginglymus)* has one axis, one degree of freedom, e.g., the phalanges of the fingers
2. the rotating joint *(articulatio trochoidea)* has one axis, one degree of freedom, e.g., the joint between radius and ulna
3. saddle-shaped joint *(articulatio sellaris):* two axes, two degrees of freedom, e.g., between carpus and metacarpus
4. egg-shaped joint *(articulatio ellipsoidea):* two axes, two degrees of freedom, e.g., the joint between ulna and carpus
5. ball-shaped joint *(articulatio spheroidea):* three axes, three degrees of freedom, e.g., the hip and shoulder joints

The foremost directions of the movement of bones in a joint have been classified:

abduction	— away from the median line (in the frontal plane)
adduction	— toward the median line (in the frontal plane)
anteflexion	— forward (in the sagittal plane)
retroflexion or *extension*	— backward (in the sagittal plane)
endorotation	— inward rotation
exorotation	— outward rotation

Hence, a muscle that moves a bone away from the body midline is called an *abductor,* while one that draws the bone toward the midline is an *adductor.* A muscle causing bending is a *flexor,* and its antagonist an *extensor* or stretcher. The muscles engaged in exo- and endorotation are called *exorotators* and *endorotators,* respectively, mediating outward and inward rotation.

In the hand, we distinguish between *ulnar* and *radial abduction* and between *palmar* and *dorsal flexion,* while in the feet we have *tibial* and *fibular abduction* and *plantar* and *dorsal flexion.*

THE JAW JOINT

The heads of the lower jaw are hinged in the mandibular fossa of the temporal bone (temporomandibular articulation). Freedom of mobility is increased by a cartilaginous disc which, at the same time, divides the joint into two compartments. The stability of the mandibular joint depends mainly on the surrounding muscles. The opening of the mouth (depression of the lower jaw) is performed by the lateral pterygoid muscle and the digastric muscle, whereas the effect of gravitation is counteracted by the temporal muscle. In shutting the mouth (elevating the lower jaw), the following muscles are involved, in this order of importance: the temporal, the masseter, and the pterygoid. The lower jaw can also be pushed forward parallel to its position (called protraction) by the lateral pterygoid and medial muscles, and can be pulled backward (retracted) by parts of the temporal and the masseter muscles. All these muscles are involved in moving the lower jaw laterally.

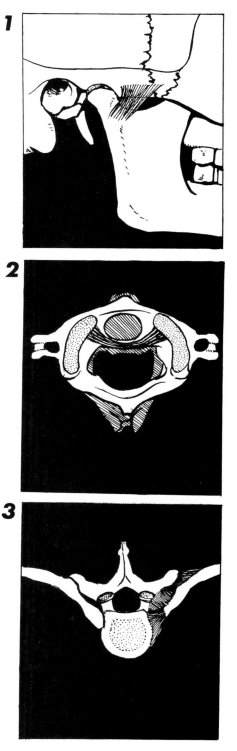

THE HEAD JOINT

The two uppermost vertebrae are formed in such a way that the first, the atlas, can rotate around a vertical process (dens) of the second one (axial vertebra, or axis). This atlantoaxial joint permits movement around a vertical axis. In the atlanto-occipital joint, the upper surface of the atlas forms a joint with the knobs projecting from the occiput, whereby nodding becomes possible. Thus the head can move freely around two horizontal axes at right angles to one another.

VERTEBRAL AND RIB JOINTS

Between the bodies of the vertebrae lie a series of thick discs of fibrocartilage *(disci intervertebrales)*, on which a ring *(annulus fibrosus* and a central nucleus *(nucleus pulposus)* can be distinguished.

The vertebrae are also in contact with each other by means of two pairs of joint surfaces on either side, and are firmly attached by a system of strong ligaments and muscles.

Ribs and dorsal vertebrae are connected by two small joints, permitting the movement necessary for respiration (inhalation and exhalation). The cartilaginous ends of the ribs are attached in front to the breast bone.

The ribs do not run horizontally forward; rather, they slant downward. The intercostal muscles (external intercostals) aid in respiratory movements. During contraction of these muscles the upper ribs move upward and the lower ones sideward, so that the thoracic volume expands.

1. mandibular joint
2. and 3. vertebral joints, showing the most important ligaments. For details see fold-out plates A and B.

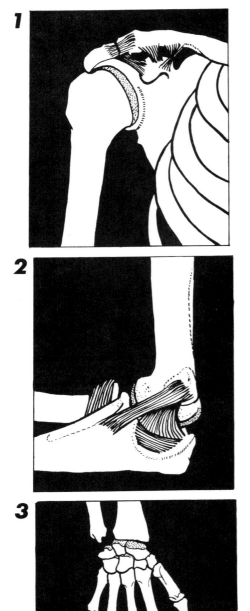

The joints and muscles of the upper limb lend a high degree of mobility to the hands and arms. The joint between breast bone (sternum) and collar bone (clavicle), the *sternoclavicular joint,* functions as a ball-and-socket joint, also through the medium of a cartilage disc. There are two articulations between shoulder blade (scapula) and collar bone, viz., between the top of the shoulder *(acromion)* and the clavicle, the *acromioclavicular joint,* and further, a ligamentous connection between the hook-shaped process of the shoulder blade *(coracoid process)* and the collar bone.

The motions that can be performed by the shoulder girdle are lifting the shoulder and rotating the shoulder inward and outward as well as forward and backward.

The *humeral joint (humerus* = long bone of the upper arm) is seated in a wide capsule fastened by many ligaments. The mobility of the arm depends also on the shoulder blade and the spinal column. If the shoulder blade is fixed, abduction of the arms is only possible to about 100°, but if the shoulder blade moves along with the arm, 155° can be reached. The stability of the shoulder blade is largely dependent on the tendon of the long head of the *biceps muscle* and the muscles in the rotator cuff *(subscapular, supraspinatus, infraspinatus).* In the ball-and-socket joint, the arm can move sagittally (abduction and adduction), round a frontal axis (anteflexion and retroflexion), and round a vertical axis (endorotation and exorotation).

The elbow joint *(cubital joint)* is composed of three simple joints: the *humeroulnar,* a hinge joint between upper arm and elbow, the *humeroradial,* a ball-and-socket joint between the upper arm bone (humerus) and the radius of the lower arm, and the *proximal radioulnar,* a rotary joint between the elbow or proximal ends of radius and ulna (the second long bone of the lower arm). There is also a distal radioulnar joint between the lower ends of radius and ulna containing a fibrous disc. Movements of the two radio-ulnar joints are accompanied by shifting of the contiguous joint surfaces, permitting the turning forward (pronation) and backward (supination) of the lower arm and the hand.

The lower arm can be bent or stretched by the elbow joint, with respect to the upper arm. Bending or flexion is performed by contraction of the *brachialis, brachioradialis,* and *biceps muscles,* while in stretching or extension the *triceps* and the *anconeus muscles* are employed.

Mobility of hand and fingers is provided by no less than 33 articulations. The joint of the lower arm and hand is the *radiocarpal joint;* the radius forms a joint with the boat-shaped ossicle, and the halfmoon-shaped and triangular ossicles. With respect to the lower arm, the hand can perform palmar and dorsal flexion and radial and ulnar abduction. For grasping, it is of great importance that the thumb can be placed opposite the fingers.

1. shoulder joint
2. elbow joint
3. wrist joint

Only a few ligaments are shown. For details see fold-out plates A and B.

Plaat Nr. 2000/2
Deutsches Hygiene-Museum,
Dresden

39 – 44

PLATE B

SKELETON
(rear view)

1. Os parietale
   Parietal bone
2. Os frontale
   Frontal bone
3. Os temporale
   Temporal bone
4. Os zygomaticum
   Zygomatic bone
5. Maxilla
   Maxilla
6. Mandibula
   Mandible
7. Sutura sagittalis
   Sagittal suture
8. Sutura lambdoidea
   Lambdoidal suture
9. Os occipitale
   Occipital bone
10. Processus mastoideus
    Mastoid process
11. Atlas
    Atlas
12. Epistropheus
    Axis, or second cervical vertebra
13. Vertebra prominens
    Seventh cervical vertebra
14. Processus spinosus
    Spinous process
15. Vertebra thoracica I
    Thoracic vertebra I
16. Clavicula
    Clavicle
17. Acromion
    Acromion
18. Spina scapulae
    Spine of scapula
19. Scapula
    Scapula or shoulder blade
20. Caput humeri
    Head of the humerus
21. Humerus
    Humerus
22. Epicondylus medialis (humeri)
    Medial epicondyle of the

I. Lig. acromioclaviculare
   Acromioclavicular ligament
II. Capsula articularis
    Articular capsule
III. Capsula articularis
     Articular capsule
IV. Lig. sacrotuberale
    Sacrotuberous ligament
V. Lig. supraspinale
   Supraspinal ligament
VI. Lig. sacrospinale
    Sacrospinal ligament
VII. Lig. iliofemorale
     Iliofemoral ligament
VIII. Lig. ischiofemorale
      Ischiofemoral ligament
IX. Zona orbicularis
    Zona orbicularis
X. Lig. meniscofemorale posterius
   Posterior meniscofemoral ligament
XI. Lig. collaterale fibulare
    Fibular collateral ligament
XII. Meniscus medialis
     Medial meniscus
XIII. Lig. cruciatum posterius
      Posterior cruciate ligament
XIV. Lig. collaterale tibiale
     Tibial collateral ligament
XV. Tendo calcaneus
    Calcaneal tendon (tendon of Achilles)

The pelvis is made up of the sacral bone *(os sacrum)* and the two hip bones *(ossa coxae)*. The latter are built up the iliac bone *(os ilium)*, the pubic bone *(os pubis)*, and the seat bone *(os ischii)*. The joint surfaces of the sacral bone and the hip bone have a cartilaginous mantle and are connected with collagen fibers. They have little mobility. The *symphysis* (the union of the two pubic bones) contains a cartilaginous disc supported from above and below by ligaments.

The hip bones form a deep cup, the *acetabulum* (vinegar cup), into which the head of the thigh bone or femur fits (hip joint or coxa articulation). The joint is supported by three strong ligaments: the *pubofemoral, ischiofemoral,* and *iliofemoral.* The head of the thigh bone lies deep in the cup of the joint and is a ball-and-socket joint.

The knee joint *(articulatio genus)* is a hinge joint between femur and tibia. It contains two horseshoe-shaped pieces of cartilage, the *lateral* and *medial menisci,* and is covered by the knee cap *(patella)*. The menisci are kept in place by ligaments. A number of ligaments in front as well as on the side and the back of the knee lend it great stability. Flexion and extension of the knee are performed for the most part by the articulation formed between the menisci and the lower end of the femur. A shifting movement also comes into play here.

Endo- and exorotation in the knee joint occur mainly in that part of the joint formed by the menisci and the tibia. The ligaments of the joint do not permit rotation when the knee is stretched.

The joints between lower leg and foot and the many joints of the foot contribute to the resilience of the body and allow the rolling movement of the foot during walking. The *talocrural articulation* (ankle joint) is formed by the fibula and the tibia with the talus. The two first-mentioned bones embrace the talus like a fork.

The *subtalar articulation* is formed by the talus and the heel bone *(calcaneus);* in addition, the talus forms another articulation with the boat-shaped bone of the tarsus. These two joints together form a uniaxial walking or jumping joint. This axis also makes inversion and eversion of the foot possible. *Inversion* is a combination of adduction, supination, and plantar flexion (lifting the inner edge of the foot). *Eversion* is a combination of adduction, pronation, and dorsal flexion (lifting the outer edge of the foot). A large number of joints are formed by the metatarsal and front portion of the foot. The pieces of bone, muscles, and ligaments are put together so that the sole of the foot is arched in two directions: lengthwise and crosswise.

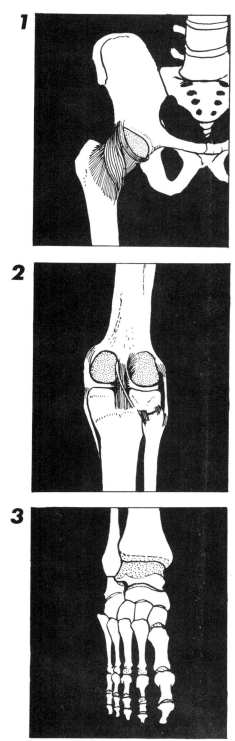

1. hip joint
2. knee joint
3. joints of the foot

Only a few ligaments are to be seen. For details see fold-out plates A and B.

MUSCLE SYSTEM

Muscles can be regarded as the organs of movement of the human body, as they have ability to contract under the influence of nerve impulses. Walking and standing would not be possible without the subtle interplay of contractions of dozens of muscles. A postural muscle is continuously "in contraction," even though there is no obvious movement.

There is a continuous-although varying-tension in the muscles that determines posture. Owing to this tension, we are able to stand or sit erect. Muscles are joined to bone and when they contract movement is initiated. Combinations of these actions form a pattern of movement. Body movements are invariably accompanied by displacement of the body's center of gravity, which, in turn, has an influence on muscle action.

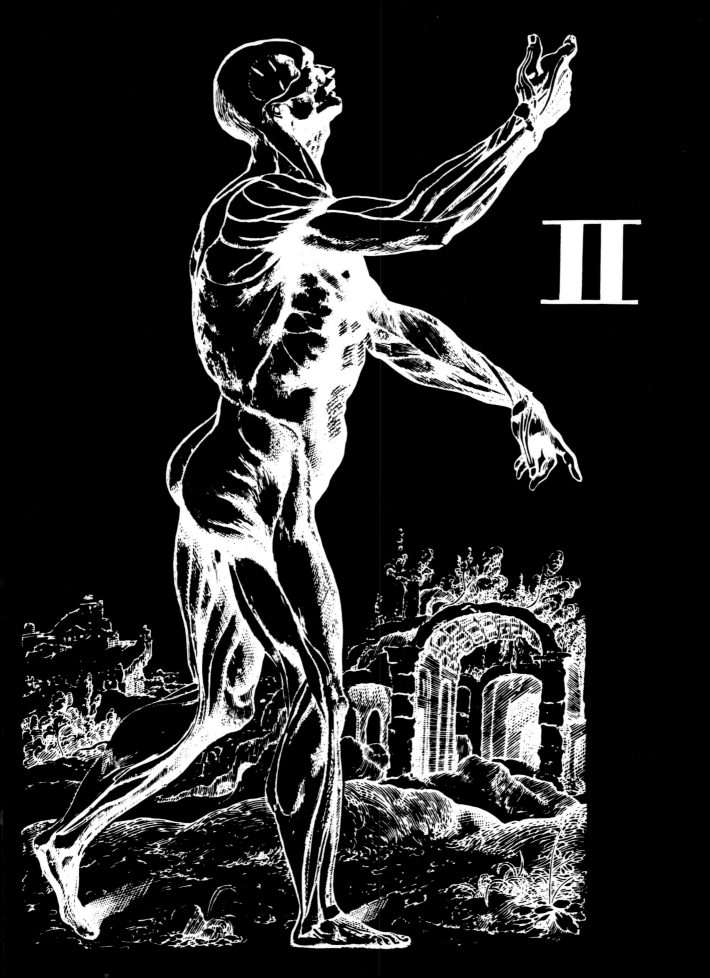

TYPES OF MUSCLES

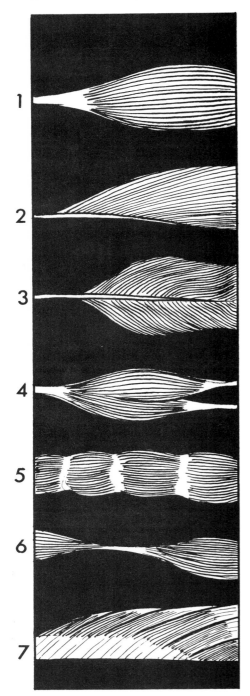

In principle, every cell in an organism is contractile. In higher animals, contractility is most highly developed in specialized muscle tissue.

There are various kinds of muscle tissue: *smooth* or *plain muscle,* found, among other places, in the intestinal walls; *heart muscle,* which consists of cross-striated muscle cells; and *skeletal muscle,* composed of multinucleate cross-striated fibers.

In man and animals, striated muscle maintains posture and provides movement. The Latin name "musculus" for muscle is the diminutive of "mus" = mouse, probably so named because of the similarity of many small muscles to the shape of a mouse. Apart from the smooth muscles, the muscular system comprises 277 paired and 3 unpaired muscles. According to the arrangement of the muscle fibers within a whole muscle, we distinguish:

a. fusiform muscles
b. pennate muscles that are shaped like feathers (pennate and bipennate)
c. flat muscles with parallel fibers
d. sphincters or ring muscles

Every muscle has one or more fleshy parts, the "belly", that contains the contractile part of the muscle, and two or more tendons connecting the belly with the skeleton or the skin. One point of connection is the *origin* or *head* of the muscle, the other the *insertion.* Muscles with several bellies are separated by one or more tendons. Muscles having several origins are called multiheaded muscles.

Depending on origin and insertion, a muscle can move one or more joints. Accordingly, there are monoarticular, biarticular, and pluriarticular muscles, acting on one, two, or several joints, respectively. Striated muscles consist of bundles of fibers lying parallel to each other, bound together with connective tissue. Thick bundles are wrapped in a very strong sheath of connective tissue, from which segments of fibrous connective tissue depart to encase smaller fiber bundles; and finally, each muscle fiber is covered with a separate connective tissue sheath. Muscle fibers are actually long, cylindrical cells that can reach lengths of 10 to 12 cm or more and diameters of 10 to 100 microns (1μ = 1/1000 mm). Each fiber contains numerous nuclei.

Types of muscles
1. fusiform muscle
2. simple pennate muscle
3. bipennate muscle
4. two-headed muscle
5. multi-bellied muscle
6. double-bellied muscle
7. muscle with large, flat tendinous insertion

Number of muscles	paired	unpaired
head	26	1
neck, nape, back	106	0
chest, abdomen	34	2
upper limbs	49	0
lower limbs	62	0

The apparatus of movement consists of the striated muscles, the skeleton, and the joints. The action of the muscles on the parts of the skeleton is partly *lever action* and partly *rotary action*. All known lever systems can be found in the human body. The following parts of a lever can be distinguished: a fulcrum = the joint; a power or force = the muscle; a weight = the skeletal part.

To illustrate the analogy of a lever system and the action of muscles and joints, three examples are given:

1. *fulcrum in the middle:* the action of the long neck muscles (m. longus colli or m. longus capitis) on the joint of the head and spinal column;
2. *weight in the middle:* action of the m. triceps surae (three-headed calf muscle) on the ankle;
3. *force in the middle:* action of the m. biceps (two-headed arm bender) on the elbow joint.

Agonists are muscles having primary action on a lever; muscles with opposing action are called *antagonists*. *Synergists* are the muscles assisting the agonists, and neutralizing muscles can act against the undesirable side effects of the agonists. The multitude of fibers of which a skeletal muscle is composed can contract in groups of various sizes upon command of the motor nerves, so that muscular action can be most accurately performed. A motor nerve cell, together with all muscle fibers innervated by it, is called a *motor unit.* The motor apparatus is aided by a number of auxiliary mechanisms to reduce friction, such as *synovial pouches,* i.e., synovial fluid contained within a membrane and located between two muscles, or between a muscle and a piece of bone, or between a muscle and the joint capsule. There are also the *tendon sheaths,* which are elongated synovial pouches enveloping the tendons of muscles.

Some Important Groups of Muscles

muscles of the head — mm. capitis
muscles of the back — mm. dorsi
muscles of the chest — mm. thoracis
muscles of the arm — mm. brachii
muscles of the hip — mm. coxae

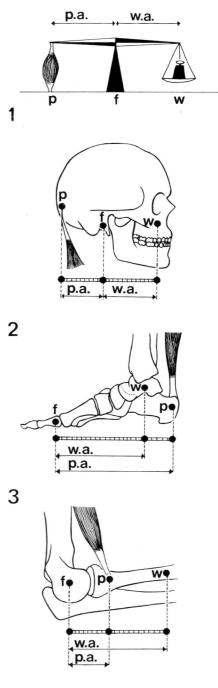

Action of the muscles on the skeletal parts

w = weight point
f = fulcrum
pa = arm of power
ma = arm of weight
p = point of power or force

1. fulcrum in the middle
2. weight in the middle
3. force in the middle

50

TABLE OF THE MOST IMPORTANT MUSCLES

The muscles are listed in alphabetical order. In the first column the name of the muscle is given, in the second column the origin, and in the third the insertion. The fourth column contains information about the innervation and the spinal level, in the fifth column the function is mentioned, and in the sixth column a test for muscle function is given.

Muscle	Origin	Insertion	Nerve supply and spinal level	Action	Test
Abductor digiti minimi (manus) (abductor digiti minimi muscle of the hand)	distal part of the pisiform, ligament between pisiform and hamate, tendon of flexor carpi ulnaris	ulnar side of base of proximal phalanx, aponeurosis of extensor tendons	ulnar (C8) T1	abduction of little finger at metacarpophalangeal joint, flexion proximal phalanx, extension of distal phalanges	supinated hand on table: abduction of little finger against resistance
Abductor digiti minimi (pedis) (abductor digiti minimi muscle of the foot)	tuberosity of calcaneus, plantar aponeurosis	proximal phalanx of little toe	tibial, lateral plantar S1, S2	abduction of little toe, flexion of proximal phalanx	—
Abductor hallucis (abductor hallucis muscle)	medial border of tuberosity of calcaneus, deep surface of plantar fascia and flexor retinaculum, flexor tendons from calcaneus and navicular	base of proximal phalanx of great toe	tibial, medial plantar L5, S1	flexion and abduction of proximal phalanx of great toe, maintenance of medial longitudinal arch of foot	—
Abductor pollicis brevis (abductor pollicis brevis muscle)	volar surface of transverse carpal ligament, scaphoid bone, trapezium bone	radial side of base of proximal phalanx of thumb, aponeurosis of extensor pollicis longus	median C8 (T1)	abduction of thumb, extension of terminal phalanx, flexion of proximal phalanx	abduction of thumb against resistance
Abductor pollicis longus (abductor pollicis longus muscle)	proximal part of dorso-lateral surface of ulna, interosseous membrane, dorsal surface of radius	radial side of volar aspect of base of first metacarpal	radial, deep branch C7, C8	abduction of first metacarpal, flexion and abduction of hand at wrist	abduction of thumb against resistance

Muscle	Origin	Insertion	Nerve supply and spinal level	Action	Test
Adductor brevis (adductor brevis muscle)	medial part of inferior ramus of pubis	upper third of linea aspera	obturator L2, L3 (L4)	adduction an flexion of thigh (external rotation)	adduction of thigh against resistance. This test is best performed with subject on his side and knees extended
Adductor hallucis (adductor hallucis muscle)	tuberosity of cuboid, third cuneiform and bases of metatarsals II and III, capsules of metatarsophalangeal joints III, IV and V	lateral part plantar surface of base of proximal phalanx, aponeurosis of long extensor muscle, tendon of long flexor muscle	tibial, lateral plantar S1, S2	adduction ande flexion of thigh proximal phalanx, maintenance of arches of foot	—
Adductor longus (adductor longus muscle)	from pubic tubercle to symphysis pubis	middle third of linea aspera	obturator L2, L3 (L4)	adduction and flexion of thigh (external rotation)	adduction of thigh against resistance
Adductor magnus (adductor magnus muscle)	inferior ramus of pubis	linea aspera, medial epicondyle	obturator (L2) L3, L4, L5 (S1)	adduction of thigh, flexion and external rotation of thigh (superior and middle part), extension (inferior part)	adduction of thigh against resistance
Adductor minimus (adductor minimus muscle)	inferior ramus of pubis, inferior ramus of ischium	adductor magnus, superior part of linea aspera	obturator (L2) L3, L4	adduction and flexion of thigh, external rotation of thigh	—
Adductor pollicis (adductor pollicis muscle)	volar carpal ligament, metacarpals II and III, volar ridge and palmar fascia of metacarpal III	ulnar side of proximal phalanx of thumb	ulnar (C8) T1	adduction and flexion of first metacarpal, flexion of proximal phalanx of thumb	to hold piece of paper between thumb and palm

Muscle	Origin	Insertion	Nerve supply and spinal level	Action	Test
Anconeus (anconeus muscle)	lateral epicondyle of humerus, capsular ligament of elbow joint	radial side of olecranon, adjacent impression on shaft of ulna	radial C7, C8	extension of forearm,	—
Auricularis anterior (anterior auricular muscle)	fascia of galea aponeurotica	frontal part of helix of external ear	facial, posterior auricular	forward movement of auricular pinna of external ear	—
Auricularis posterior (posterior auricular muscle)	mastoid process	convexity of concha of external ear	facial, posterior auricular	backward movement of auricula (or pinna) of external ear	—
Auricularis superior (superior auricular muscle)	galea aponeurotica	triangular fossa of external ear	facial, posterior auricular	raising auricula of external ear	—
Biceps brachii (caput breve) (biceps muscle [short head])	tip of coracoid process	bicipital tuberosity of radius, aponeurosis of biceps, fascia of ulnar side of forearm	musculocutaneus C5, C6	flexion of elbow and adduction at shoulder joint	flexion of supinated arm against resistance
Biceps brachii (caput longum) (biceps muscle [long head])	supraglenoid tuberosity, posterior part of glenoid labrum	bicipital tuberosity of radius, fascia of ulnar side of forearm	musculocutaneus C5, C6	flexion of elbow and shoulder, supination of forearm, fixation of shoulder joint	flexion of supinated arm against resistance

PLATE C
THE MUSCLE SYSTEM
(front view, suprefical structures)

Plaat Nr. 2003/1
Deutsches Hygiene-Museum,
Dresden

53 – 58

PLATE C
THE MUSCLE SYSTEM
(front view, superficial structures)

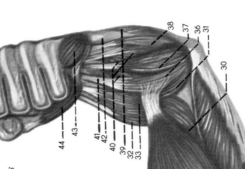

1. M. occipitofrontalis
   (venter frontalis)
   Frontal belly,
   occipitofrontalis muscle
2. M. orbicularis oculi
   Orbicularis oculi muscle
3. M. pyramidalis nasi
   Procerus muscle
4. M. orbicularis oculi
   (pars palpebralis)
   Levator palpebrae superioris
   muscle
5. M. nasalis (pars transversa)
   Compressor naris muscle
6. M. nasalis
   Head of the quadratus labii
   superioris muscle
   a. b. Pars alaris
       Dilatator naris
   c.   M. zygomaticus minor
       Zygomaticus minor
       muscle
7. M. orbicularis oris
   Orbicularis oris muscle
8. M. zygomaticus major
   Zygomaticus major muscle
9. M. temporoparietalis
   alb Superior auricular muscle
10. M. auricularis anterior
    Anterior auricular muscle
11. M. occipitofrontalis
    (venter occipitalis)
    Occipital muscle
12. M. buccinator
    Buccinator muscle
13. M. masseter
    Masseter muscle
14. M. mentalis
    Mentalis muscle
15. M. depressor anguli oris
    Depressor anguli oris muscle
16. M. sternohyoideus
    Sternohyoid muscle

17. M. omohyoideus
    Omohyoid muscle
18. M. thyrohyoideus
    Thyrohyoid muscle
19. M. sternocleidomastoideus
    Sternocleidomastoid muscle
20. M. levator scapulae
    Levator scapulae muscle
21. a. M. scalenus anterior
       Scalenus anterior muscle
    b. M. scalenus medius
       Scalenus medius muscle
    c. M. scalenus posterior
       Scalenus posterior muscle
22. M. omohyoideus
    Omohyoid muscle
23. M. trapezius
    Trapezius muscle
24. Clavicula
    Clavicle

25. M. deltoideus
    Deltoid muscle
26. M. pectoralis major
    Pectoralis major muscle
    a. pars abdominalis
       abdominal part
27. M. coracobrachialis
    Coracobrachialis muscle
28. M. triceps brachii
    Triceps muscle
29. M. biceps brachii
    Biceps muscle
30. M. brachialis
    Brachialis muscle
31. M. pronator teres
    Pronator teres muscle
32. M. extensor carpi radialis
    longus
    Extensor carpi radialis
    longus muscle

33. M. brachioradialis
    Brachioradialis muscle
34. M. extensor carpi radialis
    brevis
    Extensor carpi radialis brevis
    muscle
35. M. extensor digitorum
    Extensor digitorum muscle
36. M. flexor carpi radialis
    Flexor carpi radialis
37. M. palmaris longus
    Palmaris longus muscle
38. M. flexor carpi ulnaris
    Flexor carpi ulnaris
39. M. extensor carpi ulnaris
    Extensor carpi ulnaris
    muscle
40. M. flexor digitorum
    superficialis
    Flexor digitorum sublimis
    muscle

41. M. flexor pollicis longus
    Flexor pollicis longus
42. Ulna
    Ulna
43. M. abductor digiti minimi
    Abductor digiti minimi
    muscle of hand
44. M. abductor pollicis brevis
    Abductor pollicis brevis
    muscle
45. M. abductor pollicis longus
    Abductor pollicis longus
    muscle
46. M. extensor pollicis brevis
    Extensor pollicis brevis
    muscle
47. Retinaculum musculorum
    extensorum
    Extensor retinaculum of
    upper limb
48. Mm. interossei dorsales
    Dorsal interosseous muscles
    of hand

Muscle	Origin	Insertion	Nerve supply and spinal level	Action	Test
Biceps femoris (caput breve) (biceps femoris muscle [short head])	lateral lip of linea aspera, supracondylar ridge, lateral intermuscular septum	head of fibula, lateral condyle of tibia	common peroneal (L5) S1, S2	extension and adduction of thigh, flexion of leg	—
Biceps femoris (caput longum) (biceps femoris muscle [long head])	ischial tuberosity, sacrotuberous ligament	head of fibula, lateral condyle of tibia	tibial (L5) S1, S2	extension and adduction of thigh, flexion of leg, external rotation of leg	—
Brachialis (brachialis muscle)	anterolateral and antero-medial surface of humerus, medial and lateral intermuscular septum	ulnar tuberosity, coronoid process	musculocutaneus C5, C6	flexion of forearm, flexion of arm against resistance	—
Brachioradialis (brachioradialis muscle)	upper 2/3 of lateral epicondylar ridge of humerus, lateral intermuscular septum	lateral side of base of styloid process of radius	radial (C5) C6	flexion of forearm, supination, when arm is extended and pronated, pronation, when arm is fixed and supinated	flexion of forearm against resistance in a position which is neither supinated nor pronated
Buccinator (buccinator muscle)	buccinator crest of mandible, molar portion of alveolar process of maxilla	mucosa and skin around mouth	facial, buccal branches —	pulling of lips against teeth, drawing corners of mouth laterally aids in mastication, swallowing and whistling	—
Coracobrachialis (coracobrachialis muscle)	coracoid process of scapula, tendon of caput breve of biceps	medial surface and ridge of proximal humerus of shaft	musculocutaneus (C6) C7	adduction and flexion in shoulder	—

Muscle	Origin	Insertion	Nerve supply and spinal level	Action	Test
Deltoideus (deltoid muscle)	lateral $1/3$ of clavicle, acromion, spine of scapula	deltoid tuberosity of humerus	axillary C5 (C6)	abduction, flexion and extension of arm, internal and external rotation	abduction of arm toward the horizontal against resistance
Diaphragma (diaphragm muscle)	xiphoid process, lumbar vertebrae, costal cartilages	central tendon of diaphragm	phrenic, intercostals (C3) C4 (C5)	respiratory action	—
Digastricus (venter anterior) (digastric muscle, anterior belly)	digastric fossa of mandible	body of hyoid bone	trigeminal, mylohyoid —	retraction and elevation of hyoid bone and tongue	—
Digastricus (venter posterior) (digastric muscle, posterior belly)	mastoid notch of temporal bone	body of hyoid bone	facial, digastric —	elevation of hyoid bone and assists in opening the jaws	—

Muscle	Origin	Insertion	Nerve supply and spinal level	Action	Test
Erector spinae (erector spinae)	Three groups of muscles are distinguished: 1. spinotransverse group splenius capitis muscle splenius cervicis muscle 2. transversospinal group rotarores muscle multifidus muscle semispinalis capitis muscle semispinalis cervicis muscle semispinalis thoracis muscle 3. longitudinal system medial group interspinalis capitis muscle spinalis capitis muscle spinalis cervicis muscle spinalis thoracis muscle lateral group intertransversarii muscle longissimus capitis muscle longissimus cervicis muscle longissimus thoracis muscle iliocostalis muscle		all muscles are innervated by the dorsal branches of the spinal nerves the upper two cervical vertebrae are connected to the occipital bone with a number of small muscles: rectus capitis posterior major muscle rectus capitis posterior minor muscle obliquus capitis superior muscle obliquus capitis inferior muscle rectus capitis anterior muscle rectus capitis lateralis muscle		
Extensor carpi radialis brevis (extensor carpi radialis brevis muscle)	lateral epicondyle of humerus, radial collateral ligament of elbow joint, intermuscular septum	dorsal side of base of metacarpal III (II)	radial (C6) C7 (C8)	extension and radial abduction of hand	—

Muscles	Origin	Insertion	Nerve supply and spinal level	Action	Test
Extensor carpi radialis longus (extensor carpi radialis longus muscle)	lateral intermuscular septum, lateral epicondylar ridge, tendinous origin from some extensor muscles	lateral part of base of metacarpal II	radial (C6) C7 (C8)	dorsal flexion and abduction of hand, flexion of forearm	extension of hand at wrist joint toward radial side of forearm against resistance
Extensor carpi ulnaris (extensor carpi ulnaris muscle)	humeral head: distal part of dorsal side of lateral epicondyle ulnar head: proximal 3/4 dorsal side of ulna	tubercle on medial side of base of metacarpal V	radial deep branch C7 (C8)	extension and ulnar abduction of hand, extension and abduction of metacarpal V	extension of hand at wrist joint toward ulnar side of forearm against resistance
Extensor digiti minimi (extensor digiti minimi muscle)	lateral epicondyle of humerus	dorsal surface of proximal phalanx of little finger	radial deep branch C7 (C8)	extension of little finger	—
Extensor digitorum communis (extensor digitorum muscle of the hand)	lateral epicondyle, antebrachial fascia and intermuscular septum	four tendons into the bases of phalanges II to V	radial deep branch C7 (C8)	extension of fingers at metacarpophalangeal joints, spreading of fingers, extension of fingers at interphalangeal joints	—
Extensor digitorum brevis (extensor digitorum brevis muscle of the foot)	lateral and superior surface of calcaneus, apex of extensor retinaculum	dorsal surface of proximal phalanges I, II, III, IV	common peroneal, deep peroneal S1, S2	extension of proximal phalanges I, II, III, IV	—

Muscle	Origin	Insertion	Nerve supply and spinal level	Action	Test
Extensor digitorum longus (extensor digitorum longus muscle of the foot)	lateral condyle of tibia, anterior crest of fibula, interosseous membrane, deep fascia and intermuscular septa	one tendon to the base of middle phalanx II to V, two tendons to the base of distal phalanx II to V	common peroneal, deep peroneal (L4) L5, S1, S2	dorsiflexion of foot at ankle joint, extension at metacarpophalangeal and interphalangeal joints II to V, slight eversion of foot	dorsiflexion of toes against resistance, dorsiflexion of foot
Extensor hallucis brevis (extensor hallucis brevis muscle)	extensor digitorum brevis muscle	metatarsal of great toe	common peroneal, deep peroneal L5, S1	extension of great toe	—
Extensor hallucis longus (extensor hallucis longus muscle)	distal half of interosseous membrane, anterior surface of fibula	base of distal phalanx of great toe	common peroneal, deep peroneal L5, S1	dorsiflexion of foot at ankle joint, extension of great toe	dorsiflexion of great toe against resistance, the tendon of the muscle can be palpated
Extensor indicis (extensor indicis muscle)	distal 1/3 of posterior surface of ulna, interosseous membrane	dorsal aponeurosis of index finger	radial, deep branch C7 (C8)	extension of proximal phalanx, adduction of index finger	extension of index finger against resistance

Muscle	Origin	Insertion	Nerve supply and spinal level	Action	Test
Extensor pollicis brevis (extensor pollicis brevis muscle)	middle 1/3 of medial portion of dorsal surface of radius, interosseous membrane	base of proximal phalanx of thumb	radial, deep branch C7 (C8)	extension and abduction of thumb at metacarpophalangeal joint, radial abduction of hand at wrist joint	extension of thumb at metacarpophalangeal joint against resistance
Extensor pollicis longus (extensor pollicis longus muscle)	lateral part of dorsal surface of ulna, interosseous membrane	base of distal phalanx	radial, deep branch C7 (C8)	extension of distal phalanx, drawing of extended thumb toward metacarpal II, radial abduction of hand at wrist joint	extension of thumb against resistance
Flexor carpi radialis (flexor carpi radialis muscle)	common tendon attached to medial epicondyle, antebrachial fascia	base of metacarpal II (III)	median (C6) C7 (C8)	flexion of hand at wrist joint, flexion and pronation of forearm, slight abduction of hand	flexion of hand at wrist joint towards radial side of forearm against resistance
Flexor carpi ulnaris (flexor carpi ulnaris muscle)	*humeral head:* medial epicondyle of humerus, adjacent intermuscular septum, deep fascia of forearm *ulnar head:* medial side of olecranon, upper 2/3 dorsal part of ulna	palmar aponeurosis, pisiform bone, hamata bone, base of metacarpals III, IV, V	ulnar (C6) C7 (C8)	flexion and abduction of hand (towards ulna), fixation of wrist joint during extension of fingers (bending elbow)	hand supinated on table: abduction of little finger against resistance

Muscle	Origin	Insertion	Nerve supply and spinal level	Action	Test
Flexor digiti minimi brevis (manus) (flexor digiti minimi brevis of the hand)	transverse carpal ligament, hook of hamate bone	medial surface of body and head of metacarpal V	ulnar (C8) T1	flexion of proximal phalanx of little finger	—
Flexor digiti minimi brevis (pedis) (flexor digiti minimi brevis of the foot)	medial and lateral process of calcaneal tuberosity, long plantar ligament, lateral intermuscular septum	lateral surface of proximal phalanx of little toe, metatarsophalangeal capsule	tibial, lateral plantar S1, S2	flexion and abduction of proximal phalanx of little toe, maintenance of lateral longitudinal arch of foot	—
Flexor digitorum pedis brevis (flexor digitorum brevis muscle of the foot)	medial process of calcaneal tuberosity, medial and lateral intermuscular septum, posterior third of plantar aponeurosis	middle phalanx of four lateral toes	tibial, medial plantar L5, S1	flexion of middle and proximal phalanges of 4 lateral toes, flexion of proximal phalanges on metatarsals	flexion of 4 lateral toes
Flexor digitorum pedis longus (flexor digitorum longus muscle of the foot)	posterior tibial and crural fascia, medial side of dorsal surface of tibia	distal phalanges of 4 lateral toes	tibial L5, S1 (S2)	flexion of phalanges of 4 lateral toes, supination and plantar flexion of foot at ankle joint, support of longitudinal foot arches	plantar flexion of toes against resistance
Flexor digitorum profundus (flexor digitorum profundus muscle)	proximal 2/3 of medial surface of ulna, proximal 2/3 of volar surface of ulna, interosseous membrane	base of distal phalanges	ulnar (medial part), median (lateral part) (C7) C8, T1	flexion of distal and middle phalanx, flexion of middle and proximal phalanx	flexion of distal phalanges of little and ring fingers against resistance

Muscle	Origin	Insertion	Nerve supply and spinal level	Action	Test
Flexor digitorum superficialis (flexor digitorum sublimis muscle)	humeroulnar head: medial epicondyle, ulnar tuberosity and medial border of coronoid process, intermuscular septum *radial head:* volar border of radius, anterior oblique line	border of volar surface of shaft of middle phalanx	median (C7) C8, T1	flexion of hand at wrist joint, flexion of proximal and middle phalanx	flexion of fingers at first interphalangeal joint against resistance
Flexor hallucis brevis (flexor pollicis brevis muscle)	tendons from cuneiform bones, plantar calcaneocuboid ligament, navicular bone	lateral part of plantar surface of base of proximal phalanx	tibial, medial plantar L5, S1	flexion of proximal phalanx of great toe	—
Flexor hallucis longus (flexor hallucis longus muscle)	posterior surface of fibula, posterior intermuscular septum, crural fascia	base of terminal phalanx of great toe	tibial L5, S1, S2	flexion of phalanges of geat toe, plantar flexion and supination of foot, support of longitudinal foot arches	plantar flexion of great toe against resistance
Flexor pollicis brevis (flexor pollicis brevis muscle)	*deep head:* lesser multangular and capitate bones *superficial head:* greater multangular bone, transverse carpal ligament	ulnar side of proximal phalanx of thumb lateral side of base of proximal phalanx	median C8, T1	flexion of proximal phalanx, extension of distal phalanx, flexion and internal rotation of metacarpal	flexion of proximal phalanx of thumb against resistance
Flexor pollicis longus (flexor pollicis longus muscle)	medial epicondyle of humerus, volar surface of radius, interosseous membrane	base of distal phalanx	median (C7) C8, T1	flexion of distal and proximal phalanx, adduction and flexion at carpometacarpal joint	flexion of distal phalanx of thumb against resistance

PLATE D
THE MUSCLE SYSTEM
(rear view, superfical structures)

Plaat Nr. 2003/2
Deutsches Hygiene-Museum,
Dresden

67 – 72

PLATE D

THE MUSCLE SYSTEM
(rear view, superfical structures)

1. M. occipitofrontalis
   (venter frontalis)
   Frontalis muscle
2. M. temporoparietalis
   a/b Superior auricular muscle
3. M. auricularis anterior
   Anterior auricular muscle
4. M. orbicularis oculi
   Orbicularis oculi muscle
5. M. zygomaticus major
   Zygomaticus major muscle
6. M. splenius capitis
   Splenius capitis muscle
7. M. masseter
   Masseter muscle
8. M. buccinator
   Buccinator muscle
9. M. sternocleidomastoideus
   Sternocleidomastoid muscle
10. M. occipitofrontalis
    (venter occipitalis)
    Occipital muscle
11. Processus spinosus
    vertebrae VII
    *Spinous process of the
    seventh cervical vertebra*
12. and 13. M. trapezius
    Trapezius muscle
14. Spina scapulae
    Spine of the scapula
15. M. deltoideus
    Deltoid muscle
16. M. teres minor
    Teres minor muscle
17. M. infraspinatus
    Infraspinatus muscle
    a. Fascia infraspinata
       Fascia infraspinata
18. M. teres major
    Teres major muscle
19. M. rhomboideus major
    Rhomboideus major muscle
20. M. triceps brachii
    Triceps muscle
21. M. biceps brachii

Muscle	Origin	Insertion	Nerve supply and spinal level	Action	Test
Gastrocnemius (gastrocnemius muscle)	*medial head:* medial condyle of femur, femoral margin of capsule of knee joint, small area on back of femur *lateral head:* lateral condyle of femur, small area above lateral condyle	a common tendon with soleus muscle (calcaneal tendon)	tibial S1, S2	plantar flexion and supination of foot, flexion of knee, raising of heel	plantar flexion of foot against resistance (subject prone), the muscle should be palpated
Gemellus inferior (gemellus inferior muscle)	tuberosity of ischium, lesser sciatic notch, sacrotuberous ligament	tendon of obturator internus muscle, greater trochanter below obturator internus tendon	sacral plexus muscular branches (L4) L5, S1 (S2)	external rotation of thigh, extension and abduction of flexed thigh	—
Gemellus superior (gemellus superior muscle)	outer surface of ischial spine, lesser sciatic notch	tendon of obturator internus muscle	sacral plexus muscular branches (L4) L5, S1 (S2)	external rotation of thigh, extension and abduction of flexed thigh	—
Genioglossus (genioglossal muscle)	mental spine of mandible	superior border of hyoid bone, lingual fascia	hypoglossal	depression of tip of tongue, withdrawing of tongue, protrusion of tongue from mouth, elevation of hyoid bone	—
Geniohyoideus (geniohyoid muscle)	mental spine of mandible	greater, horn of hyoid bone, anterior surface of body of hyoid bone	hypoglossal	elevation of hyoid bone, depression of mandible (hyoid fixed)	—

Muscle	Origin	Insertion	Nerve supply and spinal level	Action	Test
Gluteus maximus (gluteus maximus muscle)	lateral portions of lower sacral and coccygeal vertebrae, back of sacrotuberous ligament, outer lip of iliac crest and outer surface of ilium, thoracolumbar fascia	gluteal tuberosity of femur, iliotibial tract	inferior gluteal (L5) S1, S2	extension and external rotation of thigh, tension of fascia lata and iliotibial band, keeps extended knee joint steady	extension of thigh at hip joint (subject prone and knee lifted against resistance)
Gluteus medius (gluteus medius muscle)	ventral 3/4 of iliac crest, outer surface of ilium between anterior and posterior gluteal lines	external surface of greater trochanter, oblique ridge on lateral surface of greater trochanter	superior gluteal L4, L5, S1	abduction and extension of thigh, external rotation (posterior part), internal rotation (anterior part)	external rotation of thigh (subject prone and knee flexed)
Gluteus minimus (gluteus minimus muscle)	outer surface of ilium between anterior and inferior gluteal lines, margin of greater sciatic notch, capsule of hip joint	anterior border of greater trochanter	superior gluteal L4, L5, S1	abduction of thigh, internal rotation (anterior part) of thigh, flexion (anterior part) and extension (posterior part) of thigh	internal rotation of thigh (subject prone and knee flexed)
Gracilis (gracilis muscle)	inferior half of symphysis pubis, superior half of pubic arch	upper part of medial surface of tibia	obturator L2, L3 (L4)	adduction, flexion of thigh, external rotation of thigh	—
Hyoglossus (hyoglossus muscle)	greater and lesser horn of hyoid bone, anterior surface of body of hyoid bone	side of tongue	hypoglossal	draws down sides of tongue, retraction and elevation of hyoid bone	—
Iliacus (iliac muscle)	greater part of iliac fossa, iliac crest, iliolumbar ligament and anterior sacroiliac ligements	femur, immediately distal to lesser trochanter	femoral (L1) L2, L3 (L4)	flexion and external rotation of thigh at hip joint with flexed leg, tilting forward of pelvis	flexion of thigh from 90 to 135° aganst resistance (subject supine with knee flexed)

Muscle	Origin	Insertion	Nerve supply and spinal level	Action	Test
Iliopsoas composed of: m. iliacus and m. psoas major					
Infraspinatus (infraspinatus muscle)	vertebral ³/₄ of infraspinous fossa, lower surface of scapular spine	middle facet of greater tubercle of humerus	suprascapular C5 (C6)	external rotation of arm, upper part: abduction of arm, lower part: adduction of arm	external rotation of arm against resistance (elbow being flexed)
Intercostales externi (external intercostal muscles)	lower margin of ribs external to costal groove	upper margin of next lower rib	intercostal T1-T11	elevation of ribs (enlargement of thorax)	—
Intercostales interni (internal intercostal muscles)	internal and external lip of costal groove	upper margin of next lower rib	intercostal T1-T11	drawing ribs together in respiration	—
Interossei dorsales (manus) (dorsal interosseous muscle of the hand)	adjacent sides of metacarpal bones	radial side of proximal phalanx of index finger, lateral and medial sides of proximal phalanx, medial side of proximal phalanx of ring finger	ulnar (C8) T1	extension of middle and distal phalanges, flexion of proximal phalanx, abduction of finger from middle finger	palm of hand on table: abduction of 2nd and 4th finger from 3rd against resistance
Interossei dorsales (pedis) (dorsal interosseous muscles of the foot)	sides and plantar surface of metatarsals, dorsal fascia of metatarsals	I and II to base of proximal phalanx II, III and IV to base of proximal phalanges III and IV	tibial, lateral plantar S1, S2	abduction of digits from 2nd toe, flexion of proximal phalanges	—

Muscle	Origin	Insertion	Nerve supply and spinal level	Action	Test
Interossei palmaris (palmar interosseous muscles)	anterior border of metacarpals I, II, IV and V	axial side of corresponding digit	ulnar (C8) T1	extension of middle and distal phalanges, adduction of fingers toward middle finger, flexion of proximal phalanges	palm of hand on table: adduction of 2nd, 4th and 5th fingers toward 3rd against resistance
Interossei plantares (plantar interosseous muscles)	proximal part and base of metatarsals	tubercle on base of proximal phalanx	tibial, lateral plantar S1, S2	adduction of digits toward foot axis, flexion of proximal phalanges	—
Latissimus dorsi (latissimus dorsi muscle)	thoracolumbar fascia, spinous and interspinous ligaments T6-L3, crest of ilium, last three or four ribs	crest of lesser tubercle of humerus, intertubercular groove	thoracodorsal C6-C8	adduction and internal rotation of arm, drawing down of raised arm *inferior fibers:* drawing downward of scapula *superior fibers:* drawing backward of scapula	—
Levatores costarum (costal levator muscles)	tip and inferior margin of transverse process	dorsal surface of rib below	cervical, intercostal C8, T1-T11	lateral inclination and extension of ribs	—
Levator scapulae (levator scapulae muscle)	dorsal tubercles of transverse processes of upper four cervical vertebrae	vertebral border of scapula	dorsal scapular C3, C4, C5	drawing upward of scapula, bending of neck laterally	—
Longus capitis (longus capitis muscle)	tips of anterior tubercles of cervical vertebrae III to VI	basilar portion of occipital bone	cervical plexus muscular branches C1-C3	*bilateral action:* bending forward of head *unilateral action:* rotation of head	—

Muscle	Origin	Insertion	Nerve supply and spinal level	Action	Test
Longus colli (long muscle of the neck)	transverse process and bodies of cervical vertebrae III to VI, bodies of thoracic vertebrae I to III	anterior tubercle of atlas, bodies of cervical vertebrae II to IV, transverse processes of cervical vertebrae V and VI	cervical plexus muscular branches C2-C6	flexion of neck, support of cervical spine, rotation of neck	—
Lumbricales (manus) (lumbrical muscles of the hand)	1st to 4th tendon of m. flexor digitorum profundus	radial border of tendon of extensor digitorum	median, ulnar (C7) C8, T1	extension of distal and middle phalanges, flexion of proximal phalanges on metacarpals	lumbricals and interossei can be tested by extension of 2nd and 3rd phalanges
Lumbricales (pedis) (lumbrical muscles of the foot)	digital tendons of flexor digitorum longus	medial side of proximal phalanx of toe	tibial, medial and lateral plantar (L4) L5, S1, S2	flexion of proximal phalanges II to V, extension of middle and distal phalanges II to V	—
Masseter (masseter muscle)	*superficial part:* anterior 2/3 of lower border of zygomatic bone *deep part:* lower border and medial surface of zygomatic arch	*superficial part:* ramus, angle and body of mandible *deep part:* upper 1/2 of ramus and lateral surface of coronoid process of mandible	trigeminal, masseteric —	elevation of jaw	—

Muscle	Origin	Insertion	Nerve supply and spinal level	Action	Test
Obliquus externus abdominis (external oblique abdominal muscle)	external surface of lower eight ribs	crest of ilium, linea alba, inguinal ligament	intercostals VI to XII, iliohypogastric T5, T12, L1	support of abdominal viscera, flexion of spine, rotation of spine toward opposite side	—
Obliquus internus abdominis (internal oblique abdominal muscle)	lumbodorsal fascia, intermediate lip of iliac crest, lateral 1/2 of inguinal ligament	aponeurosis of rectus muscle, crest of pubis	intercostals VIII to XII, iliohypogastric, ilioinguinal T8-T12, L1	support of abdominal viscera, flexion and abduction of spine, depression of thorax, flexion and rotation of pelvis	—
Obturatorius externus (external obturator muscle)	lateral surface of pubis, lateral surface of obturator membrane	trochanteric fossa of the femur	obturator L3, L4 (L5)	external rotation and adduction of thigh, fixation of head of femur	—
Obturatorius internus (internal obturator muscle)	pelvic surface of pubic rami, pelvic surface of ischium	greater trochanter in front of trochanteric fossa	lumbosacral plexus, muscular branches (L5) S1, S2	external rotation of thigh, extension and abduction of flexed thigh	—
Occipitofrontalis (venter frontalis) (frontalis muscle)	epicranial aponeurosis	skin of eyebrow	facial, temporal —	transverse wrinkling of skin of forehead, raising of eyebrow	—

Muscle	Origin	Insertion	Nerve supply and spinal level	Action	Test
Occipitofrontalis (venter occipitalis) (occipital muscle)	lateral side of occipital above supreme nuchal line; posterior part of mastoid process	epicranial aponeurosis	facial, occipital —	fixation and drawing back of aponeurosis	—
Omohyoideus (omohyoid muscle)	superior transverse ligament of scapula, superior margin of scapula	inferior border of hyoid bone	cervical plexus C1-C3	drawing of hyoid bone laterally, depression of hyoid bone	—
(opponens digiti minimi (opponens digiti minimi muscle)	border of hook of hamate, adjacent transverse carpal ligament	medial surface and head of metacarpal V	ulnar (C8) T1	adduction and flexion of metacarpal V	movement of 5th finger to base of thumb
Opponens pollicis (opponens pollicis muscle)	volar surface of transverse carpal ligament, tubercle of greater multangular bone	lateral part of volar surface of metacarpal I	median (C8) T1	abduction, flexion and internal rotation of metacarpal I	movement of thumb to touch tip of little finger
Palmaris brevis (palmaris brevis muscle)	ulnar side of palmar aponeurosis	skin along ulnar border of palm	ulnar (C8) T1	drawing of skin from ulnar side toward the center of palm	—
Palmaris longus (palmaris longus muscle)	medial epicondyle of humerus, surrounding intermuscular septa	palmar aponeurosis, fascia over intrinsic muscles of thumb	median (C7) C8 T(1)	tenses palmar aponeurosis, flexion of hand	—

Muscle	Origin	Insertion	Nerve supply and spinal level	Action	Test
Pectineus (pectineus muscle)	pectineal line of pubis, pectineal fascia, obturator sulcus and pubo-capsular ligament	pectineal line behind lesser trochanter of femur	femoral L2, L3 (L4)	adduction and flexion of thigh, external rotation (foot off ground)	—
Pectoralis major (pectoralis major muscle)	*clavicular part:* anterior aspect of clavicle *sternocostal part:* side and front of sternum, front of cartilage of ribs II to VI *abdominal part:* aponeurosis of external oblique muscle	greater tubercle of humerus	pectoral C5, C6, C7, C8, T1	flexion and adduction of arm, internal rotation of arm, raising of ribs in forced inspiration	adduction of arm from horizontal and forward position against resistance (upper part), adduction of arm from below horizontal position against resistance (lower part)
Pectoralis minor (pectoralis minor muscle)	aponeurotic slips from ribs II to V	medial border, upper surface of coracoid process of scapula	pectoral C6, C7, C8	pulling formward of scapula, pulling downward of lateral angle of scapula, aids in raising ribs	—
Peroneus brevis (peroneus brevis muscle)	lateral surface of fibula, intermuscular septa	dorsal aspect of tuberosity of metatarsal V	common peroneal, superficial peroneal L5, S1 (S2)	eversion of foot (plantar flexion of foot)	eversion of foot against resistance
Peroneus longus (peroneus longus muscle)	head and upper $^2/_3$ of lateral surface of fibula, intermuscular septa	base of metatarsal I, lateral side of cuneiform I	common peroneal, superficial peroneal L5, S1 (S2)	dorsiflexion and abduction of foot, eversion of foot	—

PLATE E
THE MUSCLE SYSTEM
(front view, deep structure)

Plaat Nr. 2033/1
Deutsches Hygiene-Museum,
Dresden

81 – 86

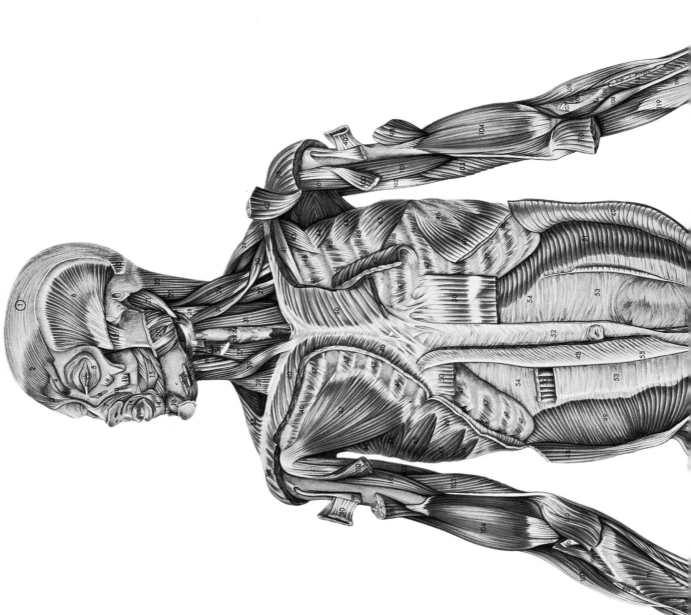

PLATE E
THE MUSCLE SYSTEM
(front view, deep structure)

1. Galea aponeurotica
   Epicranial aponeurosis
2. M. occipitofrontalis
   (venter frontalis)
   *Frontal belly of occipito-
   frontalis muscle*
3. M. depressor supercilii
   Procerus muscle
4. M. corrugator supercilii
   Corrugator muscle
5. M. orbicularis oculi
   (pars palpebralis)
   *Orbicularis oculi muscle
   (palpebral part)*
6. M. temporalis
   Temporalis muscle
7. M. nasalis
   *Compressor naris and dilator
   naris muscles*
8. M. quadratus labii superioris
   *Levator labii superioris
   alaeque nasi muscle, angular
   head*
9. M. zygomaticus minor
   Zygomaticus muscle
10. M. levator labii superioris
    *Levator labii superioris
    muscle*
11. M. levator anguli oris
    *Levator anguli oris muscle,
    caninus muscle*
12. M. temporalis
    Temporal muscle
13. M. occipitofrontalis
    (venter occipitalis)
    *Occipital belly of the
    occipitofrontalis muscle*
14. M. orbicularis oris
    Orbicularis oris muscle
15. M. buccinator
    Buccinator muscle
16. M. mentalis
    Mentalis muscle
17. M. depressor labii inferioris
    *Depressor labii inferioris
    muscle*
18. M. depressor anguli oris
    Depressor anguli oris muscle

Muscle	Origin	Insertion	Nerve supply and spinal level	Action	Test
Peroneus tertius (peroneus tertius muscle)	lower part of fibula, intermuscular septum	metatarsal V	common peroneal, deep peroneal L5, S1 (S2)	eversion and plantar flexion of foot	—
Piriformis (piriform muscle)	ventral surface of sacral vertebrae II, III and IV, posterior surface of greater sciatic notch	upper border of greater trochanter of femur	lumbosacral plexus, muscular branches (L5) S1 (S2)	abduction and external rotation of thigh, extension of thigh	—
Plantaris (plantaris muscle)	distal part of lateral line of linea aspera	Achilles tendon	tibial L4, L5, S1	raising of heel, flexion of leg at knee joint	—
Platysma (platysma muscle)	fascia over deltoid muscle and muscle pectoralis major	angle of mouth, skin and subcutaneous of part of face, lower border of mandible	brachial plexus, cervical nerves, facial nerve C7	depression of mandible, wrinkling of skin of neck, depression of lower lip	—
Popliteus (popliteal muscle)	lateral aspect of lateral condyle of femur	popliteal line of tibia, surface of shaft of tibia	tibial L4, L5, S1	internal rotation of leg, flexion of leg	—
Pronator quadratus (pronator quadratus muscle)	ventral surface of distal $1/4$ of ulna	ventral surface of radius, triangular area above ulnar notch	median, anterior interosseus (C7) C8, T1	pronation of forearm	—

Muscle	Origin	Insertion	Nerve supply and spinal level	Action	Test
Pronator teres (pronator teres muscle)	*humeral head:* central surface of medial epicondyle, overlying fascia and intermuscular septa; *ulnar head:* medial border of coronoid process	ventral surface of radius	median (C6) C7	pronation and flexion of forearm	pronation of extended arm against resistance
Psoas major (psoas major muscle)	intervertebral discs of lowest thoracic and all lumbar vertebrae, bodies of lumbar vertebrae, transverse processes of lumbar vertebrae	lesser trochanter	femoral (L1) L2, L3 (L4)	tilting of thigh at hip joint, rotation of thigh, flexion of spine and pelvis, abduction of lumbar part of spine	flexion of thigh from 90 to 135° against resistance (subject supine with knee flexed)
Psoas minor (psoas minor muscle)	lowest thoracic and first lumbar vertebrae, intervertebral discs between these vertebrae	iliac fascia, iliopubic eminence	lumbar plexus muscular branches (L1) L2, L3 (L4)	tilting forward of pelvis, tenses iliac fascia	—
Pterygoideus lateralis (lateral pterygoid muscle)	*superior part:* pterygoid crest of great wing of sphenoid, pyramidal process of palatine bone, *inferior part:* pterygoid process, maxillary tuberosity	*superior part:* capsular ligament of temporomandibular joint, neck of condyle of mandible; *inferior part:* neck of condyle of mandible	trigeminal, lateral pterygoid	rotation, protraction and depression of jaw	—
Pterygoideus medialis (medial pterygoid muscle)	pyramidal process of palatine bone, pterygoid fossa, maxillary tuberosity	ramus of mandible, lower border of external pterygoid	trigeminal, medial pterygoid	elevation and protraction of jaw, drawing jaw from side to side	—

Muscle	Origin	Insertion	Nerve supply and spinal level	Action	Test
Pyramidalis (pyramidal muscle)	body of pubis	lower part of linea alba	intercostal XII, iliohypogastric, ilioinguinal T12, L1	tenses linea alba	—
Quadratus femoris (quadratus femoris muscle)	outer border of ischial tuberosity	vertical ridge above greater trochanter	sacral plexus, muscular branches (L4) L5, S1 (S2)	external rotation an adduction of thigh	—
Quadratus lumborum (quadratus lumborum muscle)	transverse processes of lumbar vertebrae II to V, crest of ilium, iliolumbar ligament	transverse processes of lumbar vertebrae I to IV, rib XII	intercostal XII, lumbar I to IV T12, L1-L4	abduction and extension of spine, depression of rib XII	—
Quadratus plantae (*m. flexor accessorius*) (quadratus plantae muscle)	*lateral head:* lateral process of tuberosity of calcaneus, lateral margin of long plantar ligament *medial head:* medial surface of calcaneus	lateral and deep surface of deep flexor tendon	tibial, medial plantar S1, S2	flexion of toes, maintenance of longitudinal foot arches	—
Quadriceps femoris (quadriceps femoris muscle) composed of: *m. rectus femoris, m. vastus lateralis, m. vastus intermedius, m. vastus medialis*					
Rectus abdominis (rectus abdominis muscle)	xiphoid process, costoxiphoid ligament, cartilage of ribs V to VII	ventral surface of symphysis, linea alba above symphysis, superior ramus of pubis	thoracic T5-T12	flexion of vertebral column, depression of thorax	—

Muscle	Origin	Insertion	Nerve supply and spinal level	Action	Test
Rectus femoris (rectus femoris muscle)	long head: anterior inferior spine of ilium short head: posterosuperior surface of rim of acetabulum	proximal border of patella, tuberosity of tibia	femoral (L2) L3, L4	flexion of thigh at hip joint, extension of leg	extension of knee against resistance, palpation of tendon
Rhomboideus major (rhomboideus major muscle)	spines of upper 4 or 5 thoracic vertebrae, supraspinous ligament	vertebral border of scapula	dorsal scapula C5 (C6)	draws scapula upward and medially, endorotation of scapula, depression of shoulder	thrusting backward of shoulder against resistance, bracing of shoulders shows contraction of rhomboids
Rhomboideus minor (rhomboideus minor muscle)	spines of lowest cervical (VI and VII) and upper thoracic (I to III) vertebrae, supraspinous ligament, lower part of nuchal ligament	vertebral border of scapula	dorsal scapula C5 (C6)	drawing upward and medialward of scapula, endorotation of scapula, depression of shoulder	thrusting backward of shoulder against resistance, bracing of shoulders shows contraction of rhomboids
Sartorius (sartorius muscle)	anterior superior spine of ilium	medial surface of tibia, crural fascia	femoral L2, L3 (L4)	flexion of thigh at hip joint, abduction and external rotation of thigh, flexion (and internal rotation) of leg, tenses fascia lata	external rotation of thigh (subject sitting with knee flexed)
Scalenus anterior (scalenus anterior muscle)	anterior tubercle of transverse processes of cervical vertebrae III to VI	scalene tubercle on body of 1st rib	brachial plexus, muscular branches (C4) C5-C7 (C8)	raising of 1st and 2nd ribs, bending of vertebral column	—

Muscle	Origin	Insertion	Nerve supply and spinal level	Action	Test
Scalenus medius (scalenus medius muscle)	lateral edge of costotransverse lamellae of cervical vertebrae II-VII	upper surface of 1st rib	brachial plexus, muscular branches C4-C8	aids in raising 1st and 2nd ribs, bending of vertebral column	—
Scalenus posterior (scalenus posterior muscle)	transverse processes of cervical vertebrae V to VII	outer surface of 2nd rib	brachial plexus, muscular branches C7, C8	raising 1st and 2nd ribs, bending of vertebral column	—
Semimembranosus (semimembranosus muscle)	ischial tuberosity	back of medial condyle of tibia, lateral condyle of femur, capsule of knee joint	tibial (L4) L5, S1, S2	internal rotation and flexion of leg, extension and adduction of thigh, internal rotation of thigh	flexion of knee against resistance (subject prone), palpation of tendon
Semitendinosus (semitendinosus muscle)	mediodorsal facet of tuberosity of ischium	proximal part of medial surface of tibia	tibial (L4) L5, S1, S2	extension and adduction of thigh, internal rotation of thigh, flexion of leg, internal rotation of leg (knee flexed)	flexion of knee against resistance (subject prone), palpation of tendon
Serratus anterior (serratus anterior muscle)	upper 8 to 9 ribs	vertebral border of scapula, costal surface of scapula	long thoracic C5, C6, C7	drawing forward and lateraly- of scapula, aids in inspiration	—

Muscle	Origin	Insertion	Nerve supply and spinal level	Action	Test
Serratus posterior inferior (serratus posterior inferior muscle)	aponeurosis of lower 2 or 3 lumbar spines	inferior margins of the lower 4 ribs	intercostals T9-T12	drawing downward and backward of lower 4 ribs	—
Serratus posterior superior (serratus posterior superior muscle)	spines of lower 2 cervical vertebrae, spines of upper 2 or 3 thoracic vertebrae, aponeurosis of nuchal ligament	upper margin of ribs II to V	intercostals T1-T4	elevation of ribs, enlargement of thorax	—
Soleus (soleus muscle)	head and posterior surface of fibula, popliteal line and middle 1/3 of tibia, intermuscular septum	a common tendon with gastrocnemius muscle (calcaneal tendon)	tibial (L5) S1, S2	plantar flexion of foot at ankle joint, raising of heel	plantar flexion of foot against resistance (subject prone), the muscle should be palpated
Sternocleidomastoideus sternocleidomastoid muscle)	*medial head:* front of manubrium of sternum *lateral head:* medial 1/3 of clavicle	mastoid process, lateral half of superior nuchal line	accessory, cervical plexus C2-C4	bending of head and neck toward shoulder, rotation of head toward opposite side, raising of sternum (head fixed)	—
Subclavius (subclavian muscle)	first rib	a groove on lower surface of clavicle	subclavius C5, C6	depression of clavicle, keeping clavicle against sternum, aids in forced inspiration	—
Subcostales (subcostal muscles)	angles of rib	between angle and neck, 2 or 3 ribs below	intercostals T1-T11	raising ribs in inspiration	—

Muscle	Origin	Insertion	Nerve supply and spinal level	Action	Test
Subscapularis (subscapular muscle)	costal surface of scapula, intermuscular septa between it and the teres muscles	lesser tubercle and shaft of humerus	subscapular C5, C6, C7, C8	internal rotation of humerus, adduction of humerus, fixation of head of humerus	internal rotation of arm at shoulder joint (tests also teres major muscle)
Supinator (supinator muscle)	lateral epicondyle of humerus, radial collateral ligament of elbow joint, small crista of ulna	upper part of radius between anterior and posterior oblique lines	radial (C5) C6	supination of forearm	arm extended at the side: supination of hand against resistance
Supraspinatus (supraspinal muscle)	medial $\frac{2}{3}$ of supraspinous fossa, medial part of enveloping fascia	superior facet of greater tubercle of humerus	suprascapular C5 (C6)	abduction of arm, fixation of head of humerus during abduction	abduction of arm against resistance
Temporalis (temporal muscle)	temporal fossa, temporal fascia	coronoid process of mandible, medial surface of ramus of mandible	trigeminal deep temporal	elevation of jaw, retraction and rotation of jaw (posterior part)	
Temporoparietalis (superior auricular muscle)	fibers of the epicranius overlying temporal and parietal bones	fibers of epicranius overlying temporal and parietal bones	facial, temporal branch —	raises auricula of external ear	
Tensor fasciae latae (tensor fasciae latae muscle)	external lip of iliac crest, fascia lata	iliotibial band	superior gluteal L4, L5, S1	flexion, internal rotation and abduction of thigh; flexion, abduction and external rotation of pelvis; external rotation of tibia	—

Muscle	Origin	Insertion	Nerve supply and spinal level	Action	Test
Teres major (teres major muscle)	dorsal surface of inferior angle of scapula, intermuscular septum	crest of lesser tubercle of humerus	subscapular C5, C6	adduction of arm, medial rotation of arm, extension of arm	medial rotation of arm at shoulder joint (tests also m. subscapularis)
Teres minor (teres minor muscle)	axillary border of infraspinous fossa, fascia infraspinata, intermuscular septum	inferior facet of greater tubercle of humerus	axillary C5 (C6)	lateral rotation of arm, adduction	—
Tibialis anterior (tibialis anterior muscle)	distal part of lateral condyle of tibia, lateral surface of proximal 1/2 of tibia, interosseous membrane and intermuscular septum	medial surface of cuneiform I, base of metatarsal I	common peroneal, deep peroneal L4 (L5)	dorsiflexion of foot at ankle joint, inversion of foot (foot dorsiflexed)	inversion of foot against resistance (foot dorsiflexed)
Tibialis posterior (tibialis posterior muscle)	middle 1/3 of posterior surface of tibia, lateral 1/2 of popliteal line, part of body of fibula, interosseous membrane and intermuscular septa	tubercle of navicular bone and cuneiform I, cuneiform IV and base of metatarsal IV, sulcus of cuboid, capsule of naviculocuneiform joint	tibial L5, S1, S2	inversion of foot, support of foot arches (plantar flexion of foot)	inversion of foot against resistance (foot plantar flexed)
Transversus abdominis (abdominal transversalis muscle)	cartilage of lower six ribs, internal lip of iliac crest and inguinal ligament, lumbodorsal fascia	linea alba, crest of pubis and pectineal line, inner lamina of internal oblique muscle	intercostals I to VI, iliohypogastric, ilioinguinal, genitofemoral T1 to T6	support of abdominal viscera	—

Plaat Nr. 2033/2
Deutsches Hygiene-Museum,
Dresden

95 – 100

PLATE F
THE MUSCLE SYSTEM
(rear view, deep structure)

1. M. occipitofrontalis
   (venter occipitalis)
   Occipital belly,
   occipitofrontalis muscle
2. M. semispinalis capitis
   Semispinalis capitis muscle
3. M. splenius capitis
   Splenius capitis muscle
4. M. longissimus capitis
   Longissimus capitis muscle
5. M. splenius cervicis
   Splenius cervicis muscle
6. M. levator scapulae
   Levator scapulae muscle
7. M. iliocostalis
   Iliocostal muscle
   a. Pars cervicalis
      Cervical part
   b. Pars thoracis
      Thoracic part
   c. Pars lumborum
      Lumbar part
8. M. semispinalis
   Semispinalis muscle
9. M. longissimus cervicis

Muscle	Origin	Insertion	Nerve supply and spinal level	Action	Test
Transversus nuchae (transverse nuchal muscle)	occipital protuberance	posterior auricular muscle, trapezius muscle	facial, posterior auricular —		—
Trapezius (trapezius muscle)	superior nuchal line, external protuberance of occipital bone, nuchal ligament, supraspinous ligament from 7th cervical to 12th thoracic vertebrae	lateral third of clavicle, acromion and upper border of spine of scapula, medial end of spine of scapula	accessory, cervical plexus C2–C4	draws scapula toward spine, exorotation of scapula, draws shoulder upward, extension of head and bending of neck	
Triceps brachii (triceps muscle)	long head: infraglenoid tuberosity of scapula lateral head: posterior surface of humerus, lateral intermuscular septum medial head: posterior surface of humerus below radial groove, medial and lateral intermuscular septa	olecranon, dorsal fascia of forearm	radial C7, C8 (T1)	extension of elbow joint, adduction of arm (long head), maintenance in elbow in extended position	extension of arm against resistance with forearm flexed at elbow
Triceps surae composed of: m. gastrocnemius (lateral and medial heads) m. soleus					
Vastus intermedius (vastus intermedius muscle)	anterolateral surface of shaft of femur, distal $^1/_2$ of lateral margin of linea aspera	aponeurosis of insertion of vastus lateralis, proximal margin of patella	femoral (L2) L3, L4	extension of knee	extension of knee against resistance
Vastus lateralis (vastus lateralis muscle)	anterior- inferior margin of greater trochanter, lateral intermuscular septum	proximal border of patella, front of lateral condyle of tibia	femoral (L2) L3, L4	extension of knee	extension of knee against resistance
Vastus medialis (vastus medialis muscle)	linea aspera and distal $^1/_2$ of intertrochanteric line	medial and proximal margin of patella	femoral (L2) L3, L4	extension of knee	extension of knee against resistance

HEART AND BLOOD VESSELS

The blood circulation is the transport system of the human body: it delivers food and oxygen to every organ. At the same time, all metabolic waste materials produced in the body are collected by the circulating blood and delivered to their respective destinations. The circulatory blood also contains antibodies, hormones, vitamins, etc. To fulfill its transport function properly, blood circulation must be continuous throughout the whole body. Blood passes through a closed system of vessels, propelled by the contractile activity of the heart. The powerfully developed muscle wall of the left ventricle drives the blood into the large or systemic circuit of the body, while the thinner walled muscle of the right ventricle propels the blood into the shorter circuit through the lungs. A considerable portion (2000 to 3000 liters per day) of the fluid content of the thin walled capillaries located between arteries and veins diffuses from these vessels into the tissue spaces, where its composition changes and it is later reabsorbed into the circulation.

Another function of the circulation is to transport the heat produced by the muscles of the rest of the body.

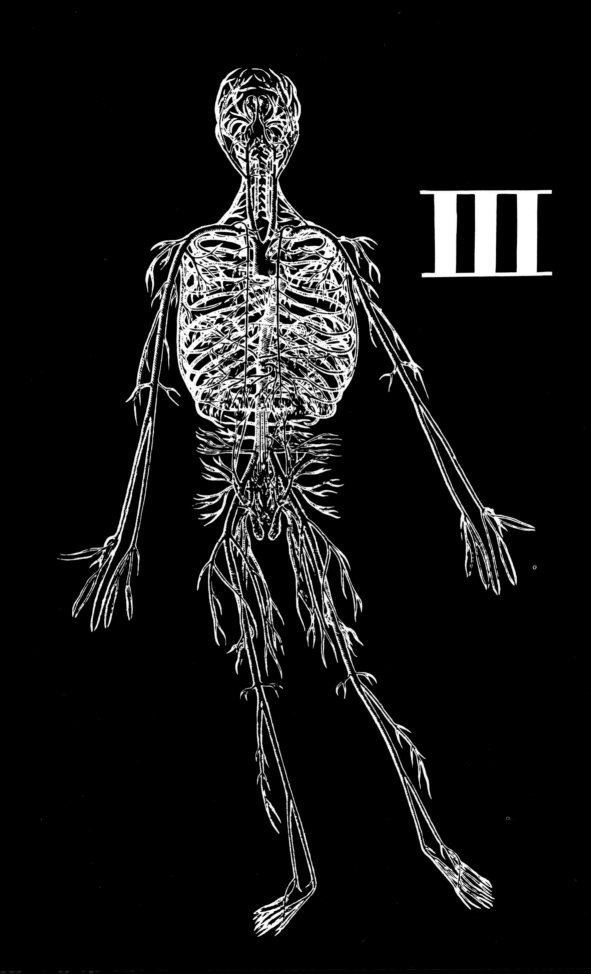

III

STRUCTURE OF THE BLOOD VESSELS

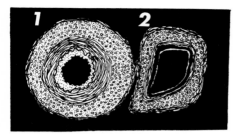

Cross sectional view of an artery (1) and of a vein (2)

The wall of an artery is composed of three distinct layers. The innermost layer, the *tunica intima,* is composed of a sheet of endothelial cells lying in a thin layer of connective tissue. The *tunica media* consists mainly of smooth muscle tissue and elastic fibers. The outer layer, the *tunica adventitia,* is primarily connective tissue. Capillaries are tubes formed of endothelial cells with an external basement membrane,

The wall of a vein is generally thinner than the wall of an arterial vessel, and its lumen is much wider, owing to its thinner tunica media. The largest artery, the aorta, has a diameter of about 3 cm, and is regionally described as follows: the ascending aorta *(aorta ascendens),* aortic arch *(arcus aortae),* descending aorta *(aorta descendens),* thoracic aorta *(aorta thoracica),* and abdominal aorta *(aorta abdominalis).*

The aorta distributes blood to neck and head, upper and lower limbs, and internal organs.

diameter of the aorta	30 mm
diameter of a large vein (caval vein)	20 mm
diameter of a capillary	0.01 mm (approx.)
length of the capillaries	3000 km (approx.)

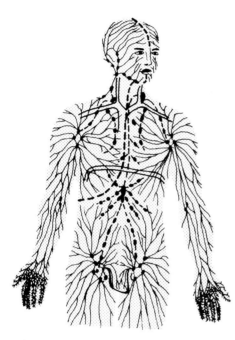

Distribution of the lymphatic vessels and the lymphatic nodes throughout the human body

LYMPHATIC SYSTEM

Fluid located in the tissue spaces is carried into the blood circulation by means of a second system of vessels. This is the lymphatic system. Its capillaries admit this interstitial fluid and convey it through increasingly larger vessels to the thoracic lymph vessel, dorsally located in the thorax, from which it is eventually discharged into the left internal jugular or subclavian vein in the root of the neck.

There are lymph nodes in various parts of the body (frequently erroneously called lymphatic glands) that act as filters, removing foreign substances from the lymph. The lymphocytes are formed in the nodes; they are counted among the white blood cells and play an important role in resistance to infection. The spleen is also part of the lymphatic system and functions as a sieve for foreign materials and, at the same time, breaks down worn-out blood corpuscles. The intestinal lymph vessels are called the chyle vessels (chylos = juice). The milky appearance of the lymph is due to the large quantity of fat absorbed from food in the intestines and carried in the lymph.

Systemic arteries take their origin from the aorta. The branches arising from the aortic arch are the innominate artery, the left common carotid artery, and the left subclavian artery. The innominate or brachiocephalic artery *(truncus brachiocephalicus)* extends upward as high as the upper limit of the right sterno-clavicular joint, where it bifurcates into the right common carotid and right subclavian arteries. The subclavian artery *(arteria subclavia)* passes beneath the clavicle in a slight curve across the root of the neck to the lateral border of the first rib, to continue as the axillary artery. The common carotid artery *(arteria carotis communis)* passes from the thorax on each side of the trachea to about the level of the upper border of the thyroid cartilage, where it divides into the external and internal carotid arteries. The external carotid artery *(arteria carotis externa)* supplies the structures of the upper part of the neck, the larynx, tongue, face, etc. The internal carotid artery *(arteria carotis interna)* enters the cranium and supplies the brain and the structures contained in the orbit. The venous blood of the cranium and part of the face is collected by the internal jugular vein *(vena jugularis interna)*. The external jugular vein *(vena jugularis externa)* collects blood from the face and the neck. The blood of both veins is carried by the innominate vein.

BLOOD VESSELS OF THE ARM

The axillary artery *(arteria axillaris)* is continuous with the subclavian above and the brachial below. The brachial *(arteria brachialis)* extends from the lower border of the teres major to a little below the center of the crease at the bend of the elbow, where it divides, opposite the neck of the radius, into the radial and ulnar arteries. Branches are given off during its course in the upper arm.
The branches of the ulnar and radial arteries form a superficial and a deep volar arch in the hand. The ulnar artery, on entering the palm of the hand, divides into a superficial and a deep branch. The superficial branch usually forms the superficial volar arch *(arcus palmaris superficialis)*. The deep branch of the ulnar artery passes into the palm between the abductor muscle and the short flexor muscle of the little finger *(flexor digiti quinti brevis)*, and joins the radial artery to complete the deep volar *(arcus palmaris profundus)*. The deep veins of the upper extremity accompany their corresponding arteries. Distal to the axilla, each artery is accompanied by two veins. The superficial veins *(vena basilica* and *vena cephalica)* run their own course. The axillary vein *(vena axillaris)* is a large vessel, conveying all the blood leaving the upper extremity.

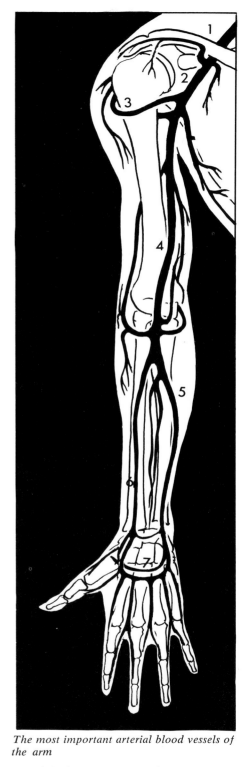

The most important arterial blood vessels of the arm

1. subclavian	5. ulnar
2. axillary	6. radial
3. circumflex	7. arterial arch of
4. brachial	the hand

THORACIC AND ABDOMINAL VESSELS

The thoracic aorta supplies many branches to the lungs, pericardium, thoracic wall, mediastinum, and diaphragm *(hiatus diaphragmaticus)*. After it passes through the diaphragm, it is renamed the abdominal aorta *(aorta abdominalis)*. The parietal branches of the abdominal aorta are distributed to the abdominal walls. The visceral branches supply the viscera. Three of these arteries are unpaired and arise from the front of the aorta: the celiac *(arteria coeliaca),* the superior mesenteric *(arteria mesenterica superior),* and the inferior mesenteric *(arteria mesenterica inferior);* and three are given off in pairs: the two middle suprarenal arteries, the two renal arteries, and the two arteries to the gonads.

The terminal branches are the middle sacral and the right and left common iliac arteries. The common iliac artery *(arteria iliaca communis)* arises opposite the fourth lumbar vertebra and terminates opposite the lumbosacral articulation by bifurcating into the external and internal iliac arteries.

The veins corresponding to the inferior and superior mesenteric arteries and to some of the branches of the celiac artery do not drain directly into the inferior vena cava, but first unite to form a common trunk — the portal vein *(vena portae)*. It enters the hepatic vein *(porta hepatica)* and there it divides into a number of branches.

BLOOD VESSELS OF THE LEG

The external iliac artery *(arteria iliaca externa)* passes at the lower margin of the inguinal ligament into the thigh and becomes the femoral artery. A major branch, the deep femoral artery *(arteria femoralis profunda),* is given off the back and lateral part of the femoral artery, about 4 cm beyond the inguinal ligament, and supplies the major part of the thigh muscles. The femoral artery, contained within a fibrous sheath, runs in the adductor canal, bounded by the sartorius muscle anteriorly, the vastus medialis muscle anteriorly and laterally, and the adductor longus and magnus muscles posteriorly. The popliteal artery *(arteria poplitea)* is a continuation of the femoral artery and extends from the aponeurotic opening in the adductor magnus at the junction of the distal third of the thigh to the lower border of the popliteus muscle. The major branches are the anterior and posterior tibial arteries. The latter gives off the popliteal artery *(arteria poplitea)*. A large number of small branches from these arteries supply the foot.

The veins supplying the lower extremities are both superficial and deep. The deep veins accompany their corresponding arteries. The superficial veins lie in the subcutaneous connective tussue. They are collected chiefly into two main trunks: one, the great saphenous vein *(vena saphena magna),* lying anteromedially, and the other, the small saphenous vein *(vena saphena parva),* posterolaterally. All the venous blood is collected by the femoral vein *vena femoralis),* which continues as the internal iliac vein *(vena iliaca interna)*.

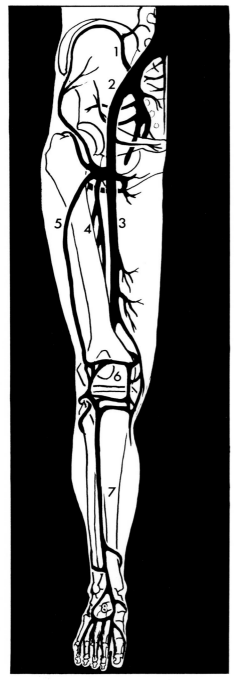

The most important arterial blood vessels in the leg

1. deep iliac circumflex
2. external iliac
3. femoral
4. deep femoral
5. lateral femoral circumflex
6. genicular
7. anterior tibial
8. arcuate

TABLE OF ARTERIES

The most important arteries of the body are listed in alphabetical order. In the first column the name is given, in the second column the origin of the vessel, in the third column its most important branches, and in the fourth column its area of supply.

Artery	Origin	Branches	Distribution
Aorta abdominalis (abdominal artery)	continuation of thoracic aorta	inferior phrenic, middle suprarenal, lumbar, celiac, superior mesenteric, inferior mesenteric, renal, testicular, ovarian, common iliacs, middle sacral	abdominal viscera and wall, pelvis, lower limbs
Aorta descendens (*aorta thoracica*) (thoracic artery)	aortic arch	bronchial, esophageal, pericardial, mediastinal, posterior intercostal, superior phrenic, subcostal	thorax, thoracic viscera, spinal cord and membranes, vertebral column, upper part of abdominal wall
Axillaris (axillary artery)	subclavian	highest thoracic, thoracoacromial, lateral thoracic, subscapular, posterior humeral circumflex, anterior humeral circumflex	upper extremity, axilla, chest, shoulder
Basilaris (basilar artery)	vertebral	pontine, anterior inferior cerebellar, superior cerebellar	brain stem, internal ear, cerebellum, posterior column
Brachialis (brachial artery)	axillary	deep brachial, superior ulnar collateral, inferior ulnar collateral	shoulder, arm, forearm, hand
Carotis communis (common carotid artery)	innominate (right), arch of aorta (left)	external carotid, internal carotid	see individual branches
Carotis externa (external carotid artery)	common carotid	superior thyroid, ascending pharyngeal, lingual, facial, occipital, posterior auricular, superficial temporal, maxillary	neck, face, skull

108

Artery	Origin	Branches	Distribution
Carotis interna (internal carotid artery)	common carotid	ophthalmic, posterior communicating, anterior choroidal, anterior cerebral, middle cerebral	middle ear, brain, pituitary, orbit, choroid plexus of lateral ventricle
Cerebri anterior (anterior cerebral artery)	internal carotid	anterior communicating, cortical, central	frontal lobe, medial surface of cerebrum, corpus callosum
Cerebri media (middle cerebral artery)	internal carotid	cortical, central	lateral surface of cerebrum and basal ganglia
Cerebri posterior (posterior cerebral artery)	basilar	cortical, central, anterior choroidal	occipital and temporal lobes, basal ganglia, choroid plexus of lateral ventricle
Circumflexa ilium profunda (deep iliac circumflex artery)	external iliac	ascending	abdominal muscles
Coeliaca (celiac artery)	abdominal aorta	common hepatic, splenic, left gastric	stomach, spleen and gallbladder; part of pancreas and duodenum
Coronaria (coronary artery)	ascending aorta	right coronary, right interventricular, left coronary, left interventricular, circumflex	heart muscle
Dorsalis pedis (dorsal artery of foot)	anterior tibial	lateral tarsal, medial tarsal, arcuate	dorsum of foot, toes
Facialis (facial artery)	external carotid	ascending palatine, submental, inferior labial, superior labial, angular	face

HEART AND BLOOD VESSELS

Plaat Nr. 2004
Deutsches Hygiene-Museum,
Dresden

109 – 114

PLATE G
HEART AND BLOOD VESSELS

HEART

1. Ventriculus sinister
   Left ventricle
2. Ventriculus dexter
   Right ventricle
3. Apex cordis
   Apex of the heart
4. Sulcus interventricularis
   Anterior interventricular groove
5. Atrium sinistrum
   Left atrium
6. Auricula sinistra
   Left auricle
7. Atrium dextrum
   Right atrium
8. Auricula dextra
   Right auricle

ARTERIES

1. A. pulmonalis
   Pulmonary artery
2. Aorta ascendens
   Ascending aorta
3. Arcus aortae
   Aortic arch
4. Truncus brachiocephalicus
   Brachiocephalic trunk (Innominate artery)
5. A. carotis communis sinistra
   Left common carotid artery
6. A. subclavia sinistra
   Left subclavian artery
7. A. vertebralis
   Vertebral artery
8. A. transversa colli (R. superficialis)
   Superficial cervical artery
9. A. cervicalis ascendens
   Ascending cervical artery
10. A. carotis communis sinistra
    Left common carotid artery
11. A. thyroidea superior
    Superior thyroid artery
12. A. carotis interna
    Internal carotid artery
13. A. carotis externa
    External carotid artery
14. A. lingualis
    Lingual artery

60. A. genu inferior medialis
    Medial inferior genicular artery
61. A. tibialis posterior
    Posterior tibial artery
62. A. dorsalis pedis
    Dorsal artery of the foot
63. A. tarsea lateralis
    Lateral tarsal artery
64. A. arcuata
    Arcuate artery
65. Aa. metatarsea dorsales
    Dorsal interosseous arteries of the foot

VEINS

1. V. pulmonalis sinistra
   Left pulmonary vein
2. V. cava superior
   Superior vena cava
3. V. brachiocephalica sinistra
   Left innominate vein
4. V. brachiocephalica dextra
   Right innominate vein
5. V. jugularis interna
   Internal jugular vein
6. V. jugularis externa
   External jugular vein
7. V. suprascapularis
   Suprascapular vein
8. V. transversa colli
   Transverse cervical vein
9. V. cervicalis profunda
   Deep cervical vein
10. V. thyroidea superior
    Superior thyroid vein
11. V. facialis
    Common facial vein
12. V. labialis inferior
    Inferior labial vein
13. V. facialis anterior
    Anterior facial vein
14. V. labialis superior
    Superior labial vein
15. V. nasalis externa
    External nasal vein
16. V. supratrochlearis
    Frontal vein
17. V. cervicalis profunda
    Deep cervical vein

45. V. iliaca communis
    Common iliac vein
46. V. sacralis mediana
    Median sacral vein
47. V. iliaca externa
    External iliac vein
48. V. iliaca interna
    Internal iliac vein
49. V. femoralis
    Femoral vein
50. V. circumflexa ilium profunda
    Deep circumflex iliac vein
51. V. circumflexa ilium superficialis
    Superficial circumflex iliac vein
52. Vv. pudendae externae
    External pudendal vein
53. Vv. circumflexae femoris laterales
    Lateral circumflex vein of the thigh
54. R. ascendens
    Ascending branch of lateral circumflex vein
55. R. descendens
    Descending branch of lateral circumflex vein
56. V. profunda femoris
    Deep femoral vein
57. V. perforans
    Second perforating vein
58. V. genu
    Descending genicular vein
59. V. genu
    Articular branch of genicular vein
60. V. genu
    Medial inferior genicular vein
61. V. tibiales posterior
    Posterior tibial vein
62. V. saphena magna
    Long saphenous vein
63. V. marginalis medialis
    Medial marginal vein
64. Arcus venosus dorsalis pedis
    Dorsal venous arch of the foot
65. Vv. digitalis dorsalis pedis
    Dorsal digital veins of the foot

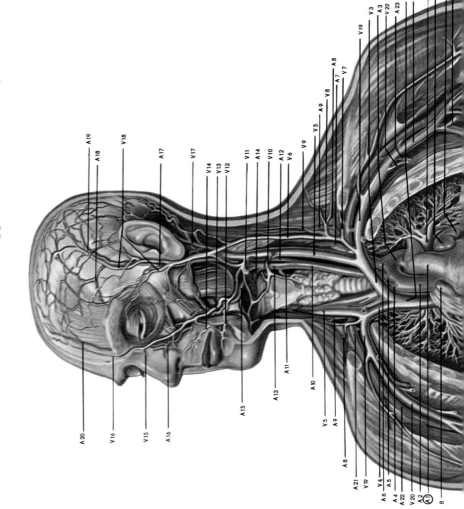

Artery	Origin	Branches	Distribution
Femoralis (femoral artery)	continuation of external iliac	superior epigastric, superficial iliac circumflex, superficial external pudendal, deep femoral, medial femoral circumflex, descending genicular	lower abdominal wall, external genitalia, upper leg
Genus descendens (descending genicular artery)	femoral	saphenous, articular	knee joint, lower leg
Glutea inferior (inferior gluteal artery)	internal iliac	a. comitans nervi ischiadici	buttock and back of thigh
Glutea superior (superior gluteal artery)	internal iliac	superficial, deep	upper portion of gluteus maximus and overlying skin, obturator internus, piriformis, levator ani, coccygeus
Iliaca communis (common iliac artery)	abdominal aorta	external iliac, internal iliac	pelvis, abdominal wall, lower limb
Iliaca externa (external iliac artery)	common iliac	inferior epigastric, deep iliac circumflex, femoral	abdominal wall, external genitals, lower limb
Iliaca interna (internal iliac artery)	continuation of common iliac	iliolumbar, lateral sacral, superior gluteal, obturator, inferior gluteal, internal pudendal, umbilical, inferior vesical, medial rectal, ductus deferens, or uterine, vaginal	walls and viscera of pelvis, buttock, reproductive organs, medial side of thigh
Iliolumbalis (iliolumbar artery)	internal iliac		pelvic muscles and bones, 5th lumbar segment

Artery	Origin	Branches	Distribution
Lingualis (lingual artery)	external carotid	suprahyoid, sublingual, dorsal lingual, deep lingual	tongue, sublingual gland, tonsil, epiglottis
Lumbales (lumbar artery)	abdominal aorta	posterior, spinal	abdominal walls, vertebrae, lumbar muscles, renal capsule
Maxillaris (maxillary artery)	external carotid	deep auricular, anterior tympanic, inferior alveolar, middle meningeal, accessory meningeal	both jaws, teeth, chewing muscles, ears, meninges, nose, palate
Mesenterica inferior (inferior mesenteric artery)	abdominal aorta	left colic, sigmoid, superior rectal	lower half of colon, rectum
Mesenterica superior (superior mesenteric artery)	abdominal aorta	inferior pancreaticoduodenal, intestinal ileocolic, middle colic, right colic	small intestine, proximal half of colon
Obturatoria (obturator artery)	internal iliac	pubic, acetabular, anterior, posterior	pelvic muscles and hip joint
Occipitalis (occipital artery)	external carotid	mastoid, auricular, sternocleidomastoid, occipital, descending, meningeal	muscles of neck and scalp and meninges
Ophthalmica (opthalmic artery)	internal carotid	central artery of retina, lacrimal, supraorbital, ciliary, ethmoidal, palpebral, conjunctival, supratrochlear, dorsal nasal	eye, orbit and adjacent facial structures
Ovarica (ovarian artery)	abdominal aorta	ureteral, uterine tube	ovary, uterus, ureter
Peronea (peroneal artery)	posterior tibial	perforating, communicating, posterior lateral malleolar, lateral calcaneal	back of lower leg, ankle, deep calf muscles

Artery	Origin	Branches	Distribution
Pharyngea ascendens (ascending pharyngeal artery)	external carotid	posterior meningeal, pharyngeal, inferior tympanic	wall of pharynx, meninges, cranium
Phrenicae inferiores (inferior phrenic artery)	abdominal aorta	superior suprarenal	diaphragm, adrenal glands
Plantaris lateralis (lateral plantar artery)	posterior tibial	plantar arch, plantar metatarsal	sole and toes
Plantaris medialis (medial plantar artery)	posterior tibial	deep, superficial	m. abductor hallucis, n. flexor digitorum brevis and sole of the foot
Poplitea (popliteal artery)	femoral	genicular, sural, articular plexus of knee, patellar plexus	knee joint and part of lower limb
Profunda femoris (deep femoral artery)	femoral	perforating, lateral femoral circumflex, medial femoral circumflex	hip joint, thigh muscles
Pudenda interna (internal pudendal artery)	internal iliac	inferior rectal, perineal, posterior scrotal (labial), urethral, deep artery of penis (clitoris), dorsal artery of penis (clitoris)	external genitalia, rectum, perineum and base of pelvis
Pulmonalis (dextra et sinistra) (left and right pulmonary arteries)	pulmonary trunk (right ventricle)	many branches to both lungs	transports venous blood to the lungs
Radialis (radial artery)	brachial	radial recurrent, palmar carpal, superficial palmar, dorsal carpal, princeps pollicis, deep palmar arch	forearm, wrist and hand

Artery	Origin	Branches	Distribution
Rectalis media (middle hemorrhoidal artery)	internal iliac	—	middle portion of rectum
Renalis (renal artery)	abdominal aorta	inferior suprarenal, ureteral	kidney, adrenal, ureter
Sacrales laterales (lateral sacral artery)	internal iliac	spinal	spinal nerves, structures about coccyx and sacrum
Sacralis mediana (middle sacral artery)	abdominal aorta	lowest lumbar, sacral, coccygeal	sacrum and coccyx
Subclavia (subclavian artery)	right: brachiocephalic trunk, left: aortic arch	vertebral, internal thoracic, thyrocervical trunk, costocervical trunk, axillary	neck, thoracic wall, axilla
Suprascapularis (subscapular artery)	thyrocervical trunk	acromial	shoulder, muscles of scapula, back of axilla
Temporalis superficialis (superficial temporal artery)	external carotid	parotid, anterior auricular, transverse facial, middle temporal, zygomatico-orbital, frontal, parietal	parotid gland, auricula, scalp
Testicularis (testicular artery)	abdominal aorta	ureteral	testicles and portion of ureter
Thoracica interna (internal thoracic artery)	axillary	mediastinal, thymic, bronchial, sternal, anterior intercostal, pericardiacophrenic, musculophrenic, superior epigastric	anterior thoracic wall, mammary glands, diaphragm, structures in mediastinum
Thyroidea inferior (inferior thyroid artery)	thyrocervical trunk	inferior laryngeal, thyroid gland, tracheal, esophageal, ascending cervical	esophagus, trachea, larynx, thyroid gland, neck muscles

Artery	Origin	Branches	Distribution
Thyroidea superior (superior thyroid artery)	external carotid	infrahyoid, superior laryngeal, cricothyroid	larynx, thyroid gland, pharynx, part of oral cavity
Tibialis anterior (anterior tibial artery)	popliteal	anterior tibial recurrent, malleolar, malleolar plexuses	lower leg, ankle and foot
Tibialis posterior (posterior tibial artery)	popliteal	—	lower leg, heel and foot
Transversa colli (transverse artery of neck)	thryrocervical trunk	superficial	muscles of neck
Truncus brachiocephalicus (brachiocephalic trunk)	aortic arch	right subclavian, common carotid	head, shoulder and arm
Truncus costocervicalis (costocervical trunk)	subclavian	deep cervical, highest intercostal	deep neck tissues and upper portion of thorax
Truncus thyrocervicalis (thyrocervical trunk)	subclavian	inferior thyroid	shoulder, lateral wall of neck, thyroid gland and adrenal glands
Ulnaris (ulnar artery)	brachial	ulnar recurrent, common interosseous, palmar carpal, dorsal carpal, deep palmar, superficial palmar arch	elbow joint, forearm, wrist and hand
Umbilicalis (umbilical artery)	internal iliac	superior vesicle, ductus deferens	portion of bladder and ductus deferens
Uterina (uterine artery)	internal iliac	ovarian, tubal	fallopian tubes, uterus and vagina
Vaginalis (vaginal artery)	internal iliac uterine	—	vagina, base of bladder, rectum
Vertebralis (vertebral artery)	subclavian	spinal, meningeal, posterior inferior cerebellar	muscles of neck, spinal column and central nervous system

THE NERVOUS SYSTEM

For descriptive purposes the nervous system can be divided into the central nervous system, consisting of the brain and the spinal cord, and the peripheral nervous system, consisting of the nerves which run throughout the body. The entire nervous system functions as a single unit, receiving and processing information. From sensory receptors it receives many tens of thousands of signals, processes these and sends back thousands of signals to the body, such as the muscles and glands. The main functions of the nervous system fall into three groups:

1. It efficiently integrates the performance of diverse organs, each directed to its own function, in a much faster way than would be possible through transportation of substances via the blood vessels. As a result, organ function is integrated to serve a higher order: that of the entire organism.

2. The individual can react in an efficient and rapid manner to changes in the external environment. The ability to adapt to environmental changes contributes to the preservation of the species.

3. Specific parts of the human nervous system must be regarded as the places where, in a manner yet unknown, the connection is made between mind and body, and where functions such as abstract thinking and consciousness are localized.

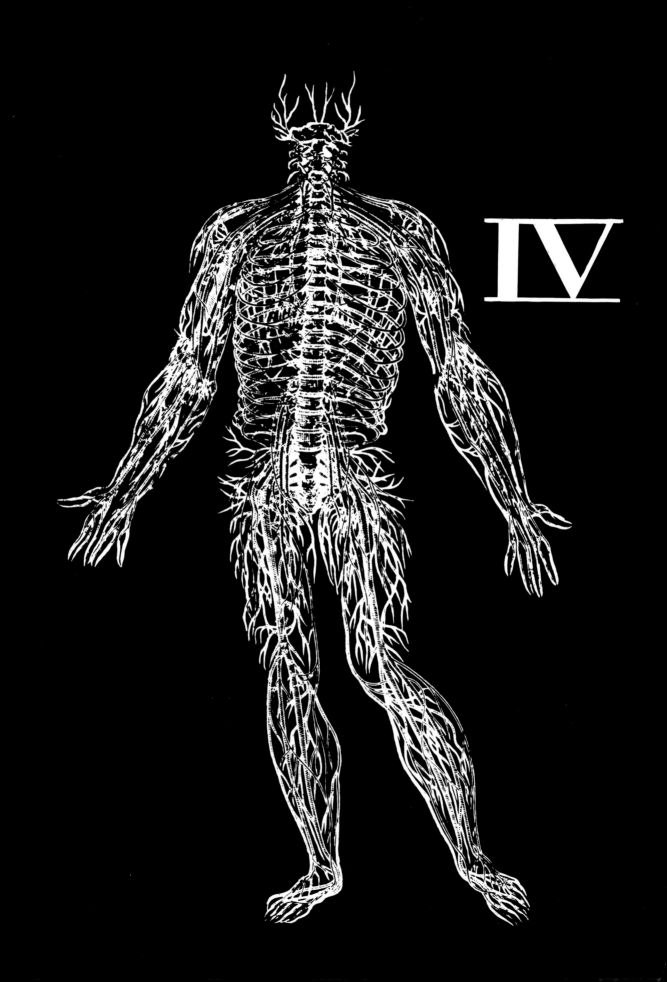

IV

THE NERVE CELL

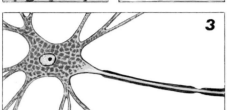

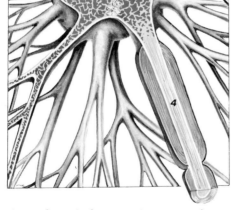

The nerve cell (3) compared with two other types of cells (1 and 2)

Most characteristic of the nerve cell is its large number of branches.

A number of the most important elements of the nervous system

1. the cytoplasm
2. the nucleus and nucleolus
3. the dendrites
4. the axon with its myelin sheath

The structural and functional unit of the nervous system is the nerve cell or *neuron.* Cells of other organs have a relatively simple shape in comparison to some types of nerve cells. The most characteristic difference is the great number of branches, which vary considerably in length. These branches are especially important in the conduction of nerve impulses or stimuli. The neuron is equipped with two types of branches: the *dendrites,* shorter, richly branching offshoots which generally receive nerve impulses, and the *axons* or *neurites,* longer, single branches which carry impulses to other nerve cells or effector organs such as muscles or glands.

The nervous system controls or regulates every bodily function. No muscle contracts, and no gland releases substances, without first being activated by the nervous system. Information from the outside world which is received through our sense organs is conducted, processed, and, eventually, brought to consciousness in the nervous system.

The workings of the nervous system, sense organs, and muscles are not independent; they are intimately related to each other. The nervous system makes possible the harmonious coordination of all organs. It is through the nervous system that the tissues and organ systems are integrated, each directed to its own function. The nervous system can be regarded as the coordinating system of the organism.

A second type of cell is found in the nervous system: the *glia,* from the Greek word which means glue, a term that was introduced in a period when it was thought that these cells were a sort of adhesive for the nerve cells. The glial cells, which outnumber the neurons, are involved in the metabolism of the nervous system, provide support, and participate in the formation of axon sheaths (myelin). The vulnerable central nervous system is completely surrounded by bony tissue (skull and vertebral canal). It consists of the following sections: *cerebrum, brain stem, cerebellum,* and *spinal cord.* The first three together are called the brain. The spinal cord lies in the bony *vertebral canal,* which is formed by round holes in the vertebrae which are linked together.

The peripheral nervous system consists of 12 pairs of cranial nerves which are connected to the brain and sent out through openings in the skull, and of 31 to 33 pairs of spinal nerves which are connected to the spinal cord and leave the vertebral canal via small holes between the vertebrae. A distinction is also made between *somatic* and *autonomic* nervous functions. The former is involved, above all, in the processing of sensory stimuli and the innervation of the striated muscles, while the latter innervates or regulates all functions related to the internal organs.

H

OUS SYSTEM
(ect)

'1

ne-Museum,

PLATE H
THE NERVOUS SYSTEM
(anterior aspect)

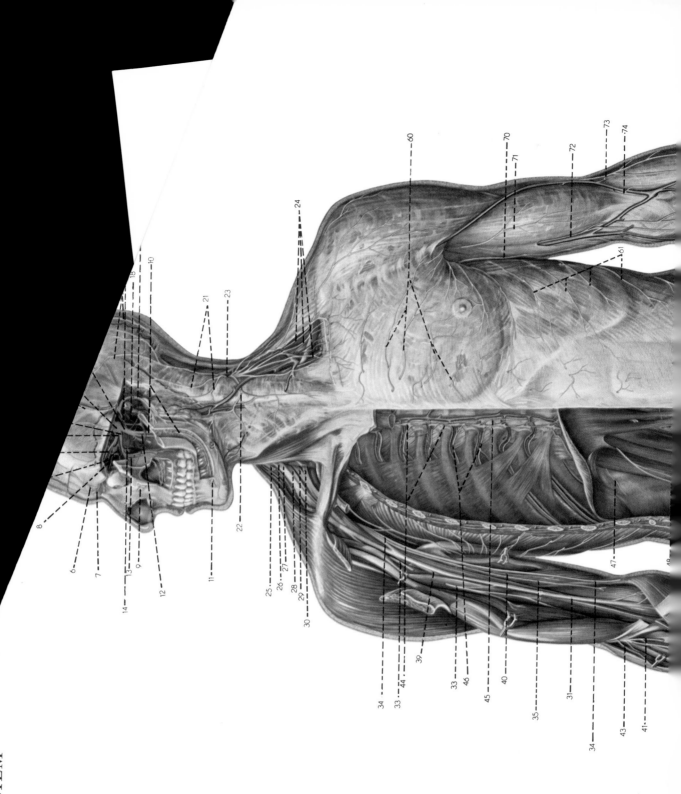

1. Ganglion trigeminale
   Trigeminal (Gasserian)
   ganglion
2. N. ophthalmicus
   Ophthalmic nerve
3. N. maxillaris
   Maxillary nerve
4. N. mandibularis
   Mandibular nerve
5. N. frontalis
   Frontal nerve
6. N. frontalis (ramus lateralis)
   Supraorbital nerve
7. N. frontalis (ramus medialis)
   Supratrochlear nerve
8. N. lacrimalis
   Lacrimal nerve
9. N. infraorbitalis
   Infraorbital nerve
10. N. alveolaris inferior
    Inferior alveolar nerve
11. N. mentalis
    Mental nerve
12. N. lingualis
    Lingual nerve
13. Nn. alveolares superiores
    posteriores
    Posterior superior dental
    branches of the maxillary
    nerve
14. Ganglion pterygopalatinum
    Pterygopalatine ganglion
15. N. opticus
    Optic nerve
16. N. facialis
    Facial nerve
17. N. petrosus major
    Greater superficial petrosal
    nerve
18. Chorda tympani
    Chorda tympani nerve
19. N. auriculotemporalis
    Auriculotemporal nerve
20. N. occipitalis major et minor
    Greater and lesser occipital
    nerve
21. N. auricularis posterior et
    anterior
    Posterior auricular nerve and
    anterior auricular branches
    of the auriculotemporal

The autonomic nervous system — also called the vegetative or involuntary nervous system — serves to regulate the functions of the internal organs such as the heart, the lungs, and the intestines. It can be divided into two more or less separate parts, both from an anatomical and a functional point of view: the parasympathetic and sympathetic systems which exercise an opposite action on the various organs. The parasympathetic division originates from nuclei of the brain stem and from the sacral portion of the spinal cord, while the cells of origin of the sympathtic division lie in the thoracic and lumbar spinal cord.

The peripheral parts of the autonomic nervous system always consist of two nerve cells linked together. The cell body and dendrites of the first neuron lie in the brain stem or the spinal cord. The axons leave the central system and run to the periphery. The second neuron originates near the spinal cord (in the case of the sympathetic nervous system) or near or in the organ to be innervated (in the case of the parasympathetic nervous system). At the point of origin of the second neuron a cluster of cell bodies produces a small swelling called a ganglion. These ganglia also contain *synapses* or contact between the first and second neurons. Located on both sides of the spinal column, the ganglia of the sympathetic nervous system form a strand, consisting of the ganglia and connecting nerve fibers. This nerve trunk *(truncus sympathicus)* extends from the atlas to the tail bone *(coccyx).* In addition to both nerve trunks, three more large ganglia are found beneath the stomach, lying in front of the vertebral column. From these ganglia, nerve fibers go principally to the stomach and intestines.

The most important parasympathetic nerve is the 10th cranial nerve *(nervus vagus,* vagus, or wandering nerve). The extensive branchings of this long nerve supply organs in the throat, chest and abdominal cavity.

The Synapse

The synapse, found throughout the nervous system, is an interneuronal connection in which the limiting membranes of two nerve cells come into very close contact. The membranes are separated by a very small space, the synaptic cleft. At the synapse, stimuli are transferred from one cell to another. The part of the synapse delivering the stimulus is called the presynaptic element and the part receiving the stimulus, the postsynaptic element. A single neuron generally receives stimuli from thousands of other nerve cells; thus, the surface of the neuron is densely covered with synapses.

The presynaptic element contains hundreds of minute vesicles (indistinguishable by light microscopy), containing transmitter chemicals or neurotransmitters which effect the transfer of stimuli from one cell to another.

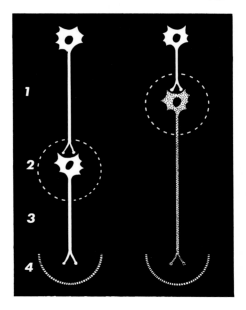

Schema of the chain of neurons of the autonomic nervous system

A. *The parasympathetic system*
   1. preganglionic parasympathetic fiber
   2. the peripheral parasympathetic ganglion
   3. the postganglionic parasympathetic fiber
   4. effector organ

B. *Schematic drawing of the sympathetic system*
   The preganglionic fiber is short and the postganglionic is long. The sympathetic chain of ganglia is located laterally and in front of the vertebral column.

THE BRAIN

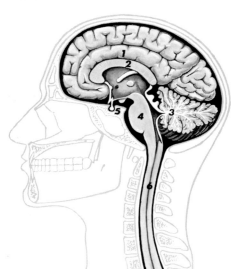

Median section through the head and central nervous system

1. cerebrum
2. corpus callosum
3. cerebellum
4. brain stem
5. hypophysis
6. spinal cord

The cerebrum consists of two symmetrical halves, the *hemispheres,* separated by a deep, longitudinal groove. The right and left halves are joined to each other by a thick bundle of fibers, the corpus callosum, and the *brain stem.* The surface of the hemispheres is called the *cortex* and consists of layers of closely packed nerve cells.

Macroscopically, the cerebrum can be divided further into different *lobes:* frontal lobe *(lobus frontalis),* parietal lobe *(lobus parietalis),* occipital lobe *(lobus occipitalis),* and temporal lobe *(lobus temporalis).* The first two are separated by a deep groove, called the central sulcus *(sulcus centralis).* Those centers which initiate volunary movements are found in the area of the frontal lobe which lies in front of the central sulcus (anterior central convolution = *gyrus praecentralis).* In the postcentral convolution *(gyrus postcentralis),* which belongs to the parietal lobe, sensory stimuli such as pain and touch are brought to consciousness. Here also is determined the function of many other areas.

The Brain Stem

In relation to the cerebrum, cerebellum, and spinal cord, the brain stem is centrally located and has a highly complex structure. On the outside, we find the white matter (myelinated nerve fibers), and on the inside, the gray matter (nerve cell bodies). We distinguish between proximal and distal regions (cranial to caudal):

a. the *diencephalon,* whose most important components are the thalamus and the hypothalamus. The latter is the coordinating center for the activities of the autonomic nervous system;
b. the *mesencephalon,* which contains the superior and inferior colliculi (centers for eye and ear reflexes);
c. the *myelencephalon,* an important region formed by the socalled bridge or *pons.* This is an important center for nerve fibers passing from the cerebrum to the cerebellum;
d. the *medulla oblongata,* which adjoins the spinal cord and has a similar organization.

The Cerebellum

The little brain or *cerebellum,* situated beneath the occipital lobe of the cerebrum, has a large number of almost parallel grooves. It is preeminent in the regulation of muscular activity.

The skeleton of the head is divided into a brain skull and a facial skull. The brain skull contains the brain and the auditory organs, while the facial skull encloses the oral cavity and also a portion of the nose cavity and eye socket.

The roof of the skull consists of a number of large, flat bones. From front to rear, they are the frontal bone *(os frontale)*, the parietal bone *(os parietale)*, and the occipital bone *(os occipitale);* the side wall is formed by the temporal bone *(os temporale)*. Further, we can also distinguish a number of smaller pieces of bone: the lacrimal bone *(os lacrimale),* the nasal bone *(os nasale),* and the vomer.

The Brain Skull

The roof of the skull is smooth and the bones are joined together in seams or sutures. The base of the skull is formed by the first four bones mentioned above and by the ethmoid bone *(os ethmoidale* and the sphenoid bone *(os sphenoidale)*. The cribriform plate of the ethmoid bone derives its name from the large number of small holes through which the olfactory nerves leave the nasal cavity. There are a number of openings in the base of the skull through which pass the cranial nerves and some blood vessels. The spinal cord passes through the largest opening in the skull, the *foramen magnum.*

The Facial Skull

The external facial skull consists of the upper jaw bone *(maxilla),* the palatine bone *(os palatinum),* the cheek bone *(os zygomaticum),* the lower jaw bone *(mandibula)* and the hyoid bone *(os hyoideum).*

Inside at the base of the skull, we can distinguish three more areas:

1. The *frontal or anterior cranial fossa,* with the ethmoid bone in the middle and the frontal bones on each side. At the rear, this groove is bordered by the small wing of the sphenoid.
2. The *middle cranial fossa,* consisting of the *"Turkish saddle",* a depression in the sphenoid bone in which the *hypophysis* is found, and the greater wings of the sphenoid and the temporal bones which together form the sides. The petrous portion of the temporal bone contains the organ of hearing.
3. The occipital or posterior cranial fossa, with the occipital bone forming the base and the petrous portion of the temporal bone forming the lateral walls.

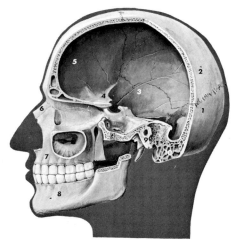

Side view of a skull from which part of the brain has been removed

1. occipital bone
2. parietal bone
3. temporal bone
4. sphenoid bone
5. frontal bone
6. nasal bone
7. maxillary bone
8. mandibular bone
9. external auditory meatus
10. mastoid process

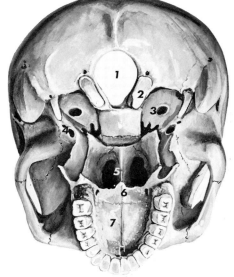

View of the skull from below

1. foramen magnum
2. occipital condyle
3. jugular foramen
4. oval foramen
5. vomer
6. palatine bone
7. hard palate

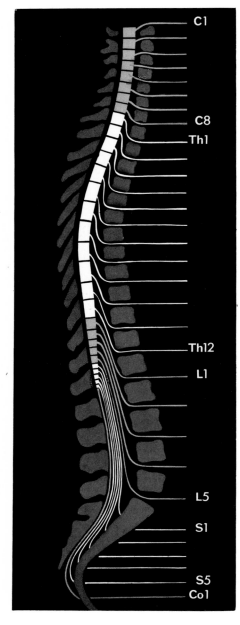

The spinal cord is a more or less cylindrical tube, the thickness of a finger, which cranially joins the brain stem and caudally ends at the level of the first lumbar vertebra. It is located in the vertebral canal, which is formed by vertebral foramina. The spinal cord has two localized swellings at the sites from which the arm and leg nerves emerge (cervical and lumbosacral enlargements). The spinal cord ends in a fine thread called the *filum terminale* or end thread.

The spinal cord is shorter than the vertebral canal and only one nerve bundle passes through each lateral opening between two vertebrae. Some of the more distal bundles travel for some distance in the vertebral canal with the filum terminale before they pass through their appropriate foramen. The filum terminale and parallel nerve bundles are called the horse tail *(cauda equina)*.

The nerves of the spinal cord supply special regions of the body. One could consider the body trunk as a structure of 31 discs stacked one on top of the other. Every disc represents a neural segment and contains a pair of spinal nerves and a segment of the spinal cord. The number of nerves which supply the numerous muscles of the upper and lower limbs influence the form and size of the segments (e.g., the cervical and lumbosacral enlargements). All spinal nerves originate from two roots; the *afferent* or *sensory nerve fibers* pass dorsally to the interior of the spinal cord, the *dorsal* or *posterior root*. The *efferent* or *motor nerve fibers* leave the spinal cord as the *ventral* or *anterior root*. While in the vertebral canal the two roots join to form a single bundle. To reach its destination this bundle will branch several times. These branches are also called nerves. Nearly all are named according to their location, the structure innervated, or by their topographical relationship. Thus, we speak of the ulnar nerve *(n. ulnaris)* because it is found adjacent to the ulnar bone.

Nearly all nerves in the body contain afferent and efferent nerve fibers. Afferent nerves carry information from sensory endings in the periphery of the body to the central nervous system. Efferent nerves carry impulses from the central nervous system to the periphery. The nerves contact muscle fibers or gland cells which are known as *effector organs*.

Schematic cross section through the spinal cord

C1 - C8   cervical segment
T1 - T12 thoracic segment
L1 - L5   lumbar segment
S1 - S5   sacral segment
Co1   coccygeal segment

The vertebral column *(columna vertebralis)* consists of 32 or more vertebrae. Each vertebra is composed of two principal parts: the vertebral body *(corpus vertebrae)* and the vertebral or neural arch *(arcus vertebrae)*. The two parts are joined by two short, thick, bony processes called pedicles. Between each vertebral body is a cartilaginous disc *(discus intervertebralis)* whose function is comparable to that of an elastic cushion. Vertebral bodies and vertebral discs form a strong, flexible column; the vertebrae provide strength, and the discs give flexibility to the vertebral column.

The dorsal surface of the vertebral bodies and the vertebral arches form the bony vertebral canal *(canalis vertebralis),* which contains the spinal cord, together with its blood vessels and the surrounding membranes. On both sides between consecutive vertebral arches there is an opening (intervertebral foramen or *foramen intervertebrale)* through which the spinal nerves pass to and from the vertebral canal. The vertebrae possess a left and right transverse process *(processus transversus)* and a dorsal spinous process that projects posteriorly *(processus spinosus).* The shape of the process varies in the different parts of the vertebral column. Thus, the spine of the cervical vertebrae is split (bifid) and points dorsally; the thoracic spine is sharp and points caudally; and the lumbar process is square and points dorsally. The projections serve as levers through which the force of the muscles can be conveyed to the vertebral column. The whole vertebral column is held together by an extensive system of ligaments (the most important of these are the *anterior* and *posterior longitudinal ligaments* which bind the vertebral bodies together) and a complex of muscles, jointly called the *erector spinae.*

The vertebral column and the back and abdominal muscles are especially important for posture. The concept of posture is difficult to describe and it is generally conceived of as the upright, well-balanced stance (of man) which is efficient and demands little noticeable effort to maintain. Abnormal deviations in the vertebral column *(scoliosis* and *kyphosis)* also directly influence stance. Scoliosis is defined as an abnormal lateral curvature in the vertebral column in the frontal plane and kyphosis is an abnormal posterior convexity of a part of the whole vertebral column in the sagittal plane.

Congenital malformations of the vertebral column are generally associated with serious disturbances in the function of the nervous system. *Spina bifida* ("open back") is a fissure in one more of the vertebral arches which failed to close during embryonic development of the vertebral canal. This malformation, as a rule, manifests itself in a deviation in the lower lumbar and upper sacral vertebrae.

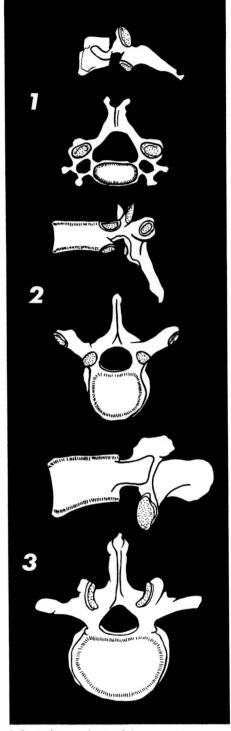

Side and top views of important vertebrae types

1. cervical
2. thoracic
3. lumbar

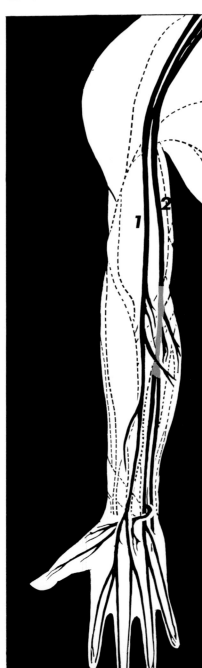

The spinal nerves from the fifth up to and including the first thoracic segment form a plexus outside the vertebral canal from which the nerves of the plexus originate. The roots of the brachial plexus pass between the anterior and medial scalenus muscles and the first rib. The subclavian artery also passes between these same structures. The most important arm nerves are described below.

n. thoracicus longus (long thoracic nerve)

This nerve runs through the medial section of the armpit, passes behind the axillary artery and then distally along the lateral wall of the chest, and innervates the anterior serratus muscle. In this nerve some spinal segmentation can still be recognized. The superior part of the muscle is innervated by the nerve fibers coming from C5, the middle part by fibers from C6 and the inferior part by fibers from C7.

n. axillaris (axillary nerve)

The nerve passes the teres minor muscle and then travels dorsally via the quadrangular space. Motor branches extend to the teres minor and deltoid muscles. The nerve continues as the sensory superior lateral brachial cutaneous nerve, which supplies a small oval area of skin at the distal edge of the deltoid muscle. It also accompanies the humeral circumflex artery, around the humerus. This is why it is also called the circumflex nerve.

n. musculocutaneus (musculocutaneous nerve)

From the upper third of the arm this nerve projects laterally, passes the humerus ventrally and perforates the coracobrachialis muscle. It continues between the biceps muscle and the brachialis muscle, near the ventral side of the elbow. The nerve supplies the biceps, coracobrachialis and brachialis muscles. Sensory branches perforate the brachial fascia and follow the cephalic vein to the wrist. The branching ends in the lower arms as the lateral antebrachial cutaneous nerve.

The radial nerve and its most important branches as seen on the ventral side of the arm

n. radialis (radial nerve)

The radial nerve is the largest nerve of the brachial plexus. Passing through the armpit (axilla) it is located between the brachial artery and the long head of the triceps. It winds around the humerus, enters the radial groove, and then pierces the lateral intermuscular septum along with a branch of the brachial artery (deep brachial artery). It continues distally between the brachialis and brachioradialis muscles and enters the forearm anterior to the lateral epicondyle, where it divides into superficial and deep branches. In the arm, motor branches extend to the triceps and anconeus muscles. The sensory branches serve the arm and forearm. In the elbow region, the radial nerve splits into superficial and deep branches. The deep branch passes between the two heads of the supinator, giving branches to this muscle and to all dorsal forearm or extensor muscles. The superficial branch progresses along the anterior lateral side of the forearm into an area bordered dorsally by the shaft of the radius, laterally by the brachioradialis, and medially by the pronator teres and flexor pollicis longus muscles. Above the styloid process of the radius the nerve turns dorsally and breaks up into terminal cutaneous branches supplying portions of several fingers.

n. medianus (median nerve)

This nerve runs superficially in the arm and follows the course of the brachial artery. In the upper part of the arm the nerve lies medial and in the lower part lateral to this artery.
The ulnar nerve also follows this blood vessel. The topography of both nerves changes when they reach the forearm. The median nerve runs from the arm to the forearm via a space between the two heads of the pronator teres muscle. In the forearm the nerve runs between the flexor digitorum superficialis and the flexor digitorum profundus muscles. During its course, branches are given off to all ventral forearm muscles with the exception of the flexor carpi ulnaris and both ulnar heads of the flexor digitorum profundus muscles, which are innervated by the ulnar nerve. A number of small muscles are innervated in the hand, and other sensory branches supply the skin of the palmar side of the thumb, index and middle fingers, the radial side of the ring finger, and the dorsal part of the distal phalanges.

n. ulnaris (ulnar nerve)

This courses through the armpit (axilla) along the lower edge of the pectoralis minor muscle, then on the medial side of the arm, medial to the brachial artery. In the elbow region the nerve runs into a groove in the medial epicondyle of the humerus and from there passes ventrally between the two heads of the flexor carpi ulnaris muscle. Superficial to the styloid process of the ulna, a cutaneous (sensory) branch is given off which supplies the skin of the little finger, the ring finger, and the medial half of the middle finger. We distinguish two terminal branches: a deep branch which innervates a number of small hand muscles and the superficial branch just described.

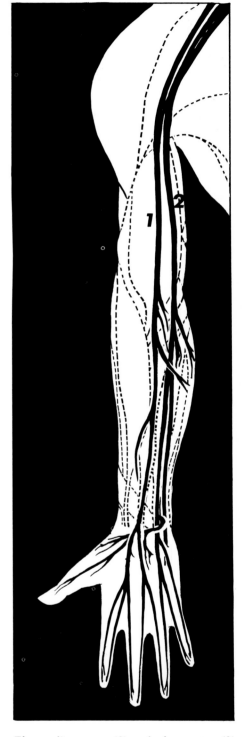

The median nerve (1) and ulnar nerve (2) with their most important branches, seen at the ventral side of the arm

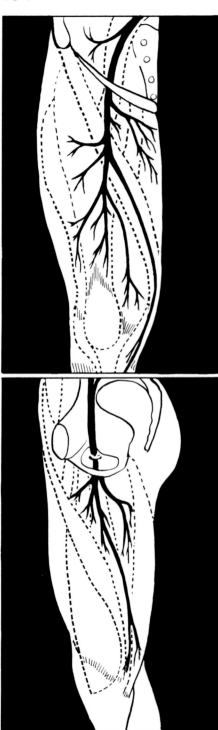

The nerves for the lower extremities originate in the lumbar and sacral parts of the spinal cord. These nerves also form a plexus outside the vertebral canal, the *lumbosacral plexus,* from which originate the various nerves for the leg. The most important nerves for the leg which arise from the lumbar plexus (L1 to L4) are the obturator and femoral nerves. The superior and inferior gluteal and the sciatic nerves originate from the sacral portion of the plexus.

n. femoralis (femoral nerve)

This nerve perforates the psoas major and appears on the lateral edge of this muscle. It innervates the iliacus muscle and then passes through the inguinal ligament, giving off a number of skin branches and also motor branches to the sartorius, pectineus, and quadriceps femoris muscles; it proceeds in the adductor canal and exits as the saphenous nerve, which innervates the skin of the medial lower leg.

n. obturatorius (obturator nerve)

This nerve passes into the psoas major muscle and emerges from its medial border. In the pelvis it passes behind the iliac artery and vein and then goes through the obturator canal. The nerve then divides into two branches: an anterior and a posterior ramus. The nerve supplies all adductor muscles and the gracilis, pectineus, and obturator externus muscles.

n. gluteus superior (superior gluteal nerve)

Coursing along the upper edge of the piriformis muscle, this nerve passes through the greater sciatic foramen and divides into two branches. The upper branch innervates the gluteus medius and the lower branch innervates both the gluteus medius and minimus muscles; it ends with a branch to the tensor fasciae latae muscle.

n. gluteus inferior (inferior gluteal nerve)

This nerve passes along under the piriformis muscle, goes through the greater sciatic foramen, and supplies the gluteus maximus muscle.

n. ischiadicus (sciatic nerve)

The sciatic nerve is the most important nerve of the sacral plexus and contains fibers from all segments, from L4 up to and including S3 or S4. The nerve leaves the pelvis inferior to the piriformis muscle through the greater scatic foramen. On the lower side of the buttock it passes between the greater trochanter and the ischial tuberosity. In the thigh the nerve divides proximal to the popliteal fossa, into the tibial and common peroneal nerves. This division can readily be distinguished even in the pelvis inside the connective tissue sheath of the sciatic nerve.

A. *The femoral nerve and its most important branches, as seen on the ventral side of the leg*

B. *The obturator nerve and its most important branches, as seen from the medial side*

PLATE I
THE NERVOUS SYSTEM
(posterior aspect)

Plaat Nr. 2037/2
Deutsches Hygiene-Museum,
Dresden

137 – 142

PLATE 1

THE NERVOUS SYSTEM

(posterior aspect)

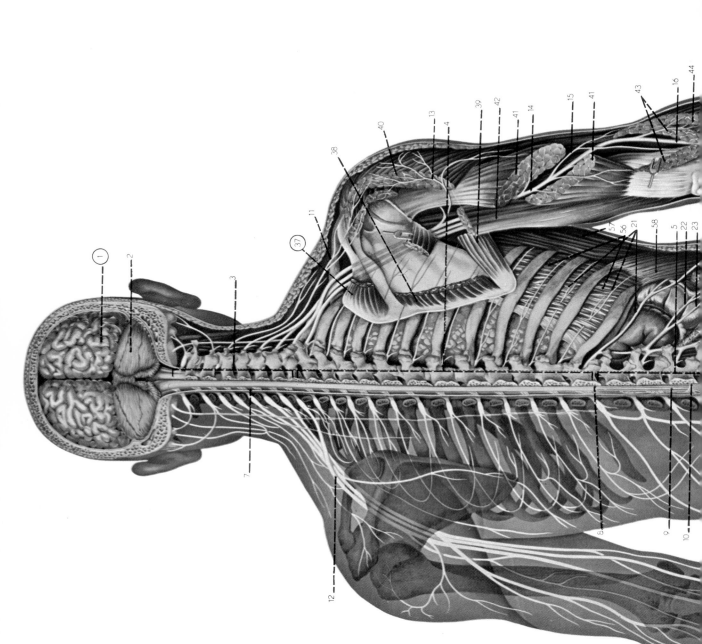

NERVES

1. Cerebrum
   Cerebrum
2. Cerebellum
   Cerebellum
3. Pars cervicalis
   Cervical region of spinal cord
4. Pars thoracica
   Thoracic region of spinal cord
5. Pars lumbalis
   Lumbar region of spinal cord
6. Pars sacralis
   Sacral region of spinal cord
7. Dura mater spinalis
   Spinal dura mater
8. Conus medullaris
   Medullary cone
9. Cauda equina
   Cauda equina
10. Arachnoidea spinalis
    Arachnoid membrane
11. Nn. supraclaviculares
    Supraclavicular nerves
12. Plexus brachialis
    Brachial plexus
13. N. axillaris
    (rr. musculares)
    Muscular branches of axillary nerve
14. N. radialis
    Radial nerve
15. N. cutaneus antebrachii posterior
    Posterior cutaneous nerve of the forearm
16. N. radialis (r. profundus)
    Deep branch of radial nerve
17. N. radialis (rr. musculares)
    Muscular branches of radial nerve
18. N. radialis (r. superficialis)
    Superficial branch of radial nerve
19. N. radialis (r. dorsalis)
    Dorsal branch of radial nerve

n. tibialis (tibial nerve)

From the popliteal fossa, the tibial nerve runs, together with the tibialis posterior artery, under the tendinous arch of the soleus muscle, through the septum between the superficial and deep flexor muscles of the lower leg, after first giving off a sensory nerve, the sural nerve, which is formed by anastomosis of the medial sural cutaneous nerve with the lateral sural cutaneous nerve. The tibial nerve innervates the flexors of the lower leg, the flexors of the foot, the long flexors of the toes (gastrocnemius, soleus, popliteus, plantaris longus, tibialis posterior, flexor digitorum longus, and flexor hallucis longus muscles). The nerve then passes medially behind the ankle to the sole of the foot, where small muscles and the skin of the foot sole are innervated. The function of the plantar surface can best be tested by various movements of the foot, such as plantar flexion of the foot and big toe.

n. peroneus communis (common peroneal nerve)

The common peroneal nerve of the leg runs laterally in the popliteal fossa, gives off a sensory nerve (lateral sural, cutaneous), and then passes under the lateral head of the gastrocnemius muscle and winds around the fibula to enter the front of the leg. Piercing the peroneus muscle, the nerve divides into a superficial (superficial peroneal nerve) and a deep branch (deep peronal nerve). The superficial branch innervates the long and short peroneus muscles, passes under the skin above the ankle, and terminates as sensory branches to the medial and middle portions of the dorsum of the foot. The deep branch passes between the extensor muscles of the lower leg, innervates them, and then supplies a number of small sensory branches to the dorsum of the foot. The muscles which are innervated by this deep branch are the tibialis anterior, extensor hallucis longus, extensor digitorum longus, extensor hallucis brevis, extensor digitorum brevis, and peroneus tertius muscles. The function of the nerve can best be tested by dorsal flexion of the foot and toes against resistance.

This nerve is one of the most vulnerable of all peripheral nerves; wounds in the area of the knee joint or fracture of the upper part of the leg (calf) can easily damage the nerve. If this occurs, the dorsal flexors of the foot and toes are eliminated, and a so-called "foot drop" results. A peroneus spring, attached to the shoe, can compensate for the handicap caused by such a nerve paralysis.

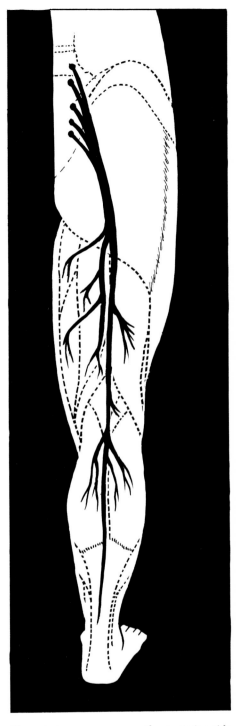

The sciatic nerve, seen on the posterior side of the leg

The nerve divides into the tibial and common peroneal nerves

THE SENSE ORGANS

The brain maintains contact with the outside world through millions of sensory cells. The stimuli which are received by the sensory receptors in both the periphery and the inside of the body reach the central nervous system as electrical signals; there they are integrated and result in conscious perception. If the stream of electrical signals from sensory receptors is organized in a particular pattern, perception or sensation occurs. This function is located chiefly in the cerebral cortex.

The adjacent woodcut, from the first edition of Vesalius' De Humani Corporis Fabrica shows the parts of the eye, our most important sensory organ.

II and III	:	front and side views of the lens
IV and V	:	the vitreous humor, with and without the lens, respectively
VI	:	side view of the vitreous humor and lens
VII	:	side view of the anterior chamber and lens
VIII	:	side view of the anterior chamber and vitreous humor
IX	:	frontal half of the lens capsule
X	:	side view of the lens, the frontal section covered by the capsule
XI and XII	:	ciliary body
XIII	:	the cup of the retina, attached to the optic nerve
XIV and XV	:	choroid
XVI and XVII	:	sclera
XVIII	:	eyeball, with exterior eye muscle and optic nerve
XIX	:	frontal view of the eyeball

SECVNDA. III.   IIII.   V.   VI.

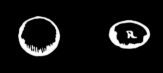
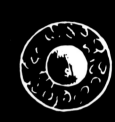
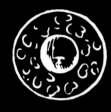
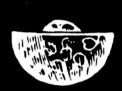

VII.   VIII.   IX.   X.   XI.

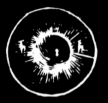
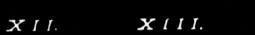
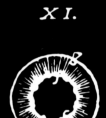

XII.   XIII.   XIIII.   XV.

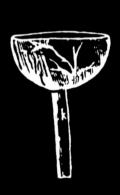
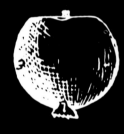
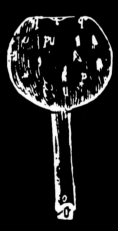

XVI.   XVII.   XVIII.   XIX.

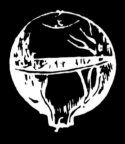
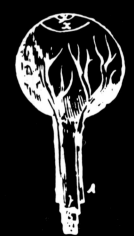
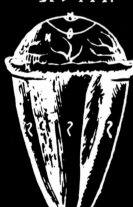
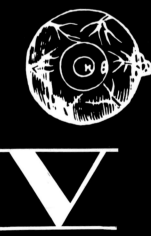

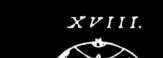
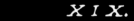

V

THE EYE

The eyes lie on both sides of the nose in the eye sockets (orbits), which are formed by several bones of the skull. The eye is a complex organ in which we can distinguish the eyeball, nerves, and blood vessels, and a number of auxiliary organs.

The *eyeball* (ocular bulb) is filled with a translucent substance and is surrounded in part by a tough connective tissue coat called the sclera, which consists of three layers.

1. The outer layer is formed by fibrous connective tissue, the white of the eye, to which the external eye muscles are attached. This layer continues forward and fuses with the transparent cornea, which has a pronounced curvature and bulges somewhat from the front of the eyeball.

2. The middle component is the choroid coat (tunica chorioidea), containing the blood vessels which supply the eye. At the point where the sclera and the cornea meet, the choroid layer becomes continuous with the iris. At the junction of these structures, the choroid coat is thickened; this is the ciliary body (corpus ciliaris), an organ rich in smooth muscle fibers. Contraction of this muscle (ciliary muscle) allows the lens to become more convex. The ciliary body extends forward to join the circular iris, in which two additional smooth muscles are situated: a dilator and a constrictor. In the center of the iris there is an opening, the pupil, the diameter of which is controlled by the dilator and constrictor muscles. The iris can have different colors, with grades from light blue to green to dark brown.

3. The third layer is the retina, which contains the light-sensitive sensory cells. This inner layer extends from the place where the optic nerve (n. opticus) leaves the eyeball to a point near the junction of the choroid layer and the ciliary body. The fibers of the optic nerve form the innermost layer of the retina; where the nerve fibers leave the eyeball no sensory receptor cells are found (optic papilla, blind spot).

The contents of the eyeball include the lens, the vitreous humor, and the aqueous humor. It is continuous with the posterior eye chamber through the pupil. The posterior chamber, also filled with aqueous humor, is located between the iris and the lens. The transparent lens is suspended by a circumferentially arranged system of fibers (suspensory ligaments) which join the lens capsule with the ciliary body. Within the ciliary body the ciliary muscle fibers can control the shape of the lens. as required for near or far vision. The vitreous humor (corpus vitreum), consisting of a jelly-like transparent substance, occupies the entire area of the eyeball behind the lens.

The optic nerve (nervus opticus) follows a slightly curved course from the eyeball as it leaves the orbit. The nerve passes through the optic foramen in the sphenoid bone to reach the base of the brain.

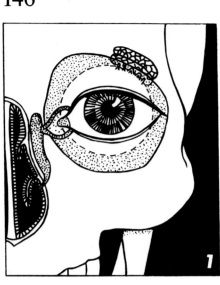

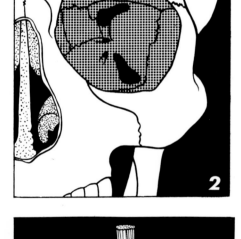

1. the tear gland and tear duct
2. the eye socket, frontal view
3. the attachment of the six eye muscles, posterior view

The organs auxiliary to the eye are the external eye muscles, the eyelids, and conjunctiva and tear apparatus.

EYE MUSCLES

Movements of the eye are determined by six striated muscles. There are four straight and two oblique external eye muscles. The four straight muscles are the upper, superior rectus; the lower, inferior rectus; the inner, medial rectus; and the outer, lateral rectus. They arise from the posterior wall of the orbit or eye socket around the optic nerve and are attached to the sides of the eyeball. The upper or superior oblique muscle runs forward from the roof of the orbit and its tendon, pierces a small ring of fibrous cartilage, which is located anteriorly, superiorly and medially and turns posteriorly and laterally to insert on the posterior half of the eyeball. The lower or inferior oblique muscle arises, on the other hand, anteriorly from the lower wall of the eye socket and then passes upward and laterally to attach to the back of the eyeball.

THE EYELIDS AND CONJUNCTIVA

The exposed surface of the eyeball is protected by the eyelids and the conjunctiva. The posterior surface of the eyelids and the front surface of the eyeball are covered by the conjunctiva, which forms a dual protective covering for the eye. The eyelids themselves are folds of skin and, with the eyelashes, they protect the eye from damage by foreign bodies. When the eyes are closed, the space between the eyeball and eyelids is completely covered by the conjunctiva, i.e. the conjunctival sac.

TEAR APPARATUS

The outlet for the tear gland is located in the above-mentioned conjunctival sac, via a number of narrow canals. The tear gland or lacrimal gland lies above the eyeball and secretes fluid in a continuous stream to this area. The lacrimal fluid is spread over the cornea by blinking of the eyelids; it keeps the cornea moist and carries away dust, and is collected in the inner corner of the eye by the superior lacrimal duct. Each eyelid contains a small opening which drains the tear fluid into and through the lacrimal sac, the nasolacrimal duct, and into the nasal cavity, where this duct finds an outlet beneath the interior nasal concha.

Some Figures Concerning the Adult Eyeball

longitudinal section	24.5 mm	weight	7.3 g
cross section	24.0 mm	thickness of sclera	0.6 to 1.1 mm
volume	7.0 cm³	cornea in section	10 to 11 mm

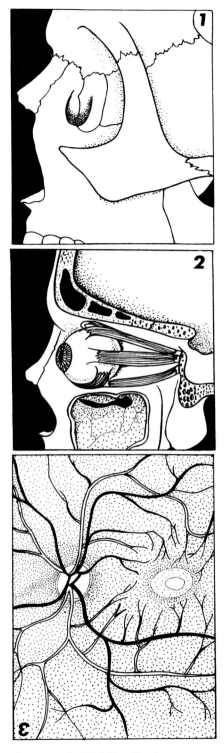

1. the eye socket (orbit), side view
2. the eye socket, side view, containing the eyeball and external eye muscles
3. the retina with its network of blood vessels

THE EAR

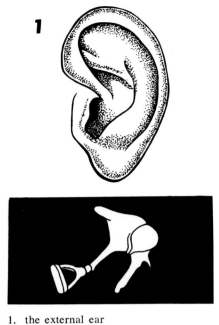

1. the external ear
2. the ear bones

The ear, the organ of hearing and equilibrium, consists of an outer, a middle, and an inner ear. The *outer ear* is formed by the auricle or pinna (a fold of skin containing elastic cartilage) and the external auditory canal or meatus, which consists partly of cartilage, partly of bone. This space is separated from the middle ear by the eardrum (tympanic membrane). The outer ear is the part of the organ which receives the sound. The auditory canal, which is partly covered by small hairs, leads the sound to the eardrum, a thin transparent membrane which begins vibrating and which, in turn, activates the ear bones (ossicles).

Small glands produce earwax (cerumen) which may plug the auditory canal. The *middle ear* consists of a tympanic cavity covered by a mucous membrane connected to a number of areas filled with air, in the mastoid portion of the temporal bone. These areas form part of the inner ear. The Eustachian tube (tuba auditiva) connects the middle ear to the pharynx and serves to equalize the air pressure on both sides of the eardrum. The three ear bones in the tympanic cavity form a chain by which the sound vibrations are carried from the eardrum to the inner ear. The hammer (malleus) lies with its handle against the tympanic membrane, and the stirrup (stapes) is attached by its footplate to a membrane of the inner ear, the oval window. The anvil (incus) is the link between the hammer and the stirrup. The *inner ear* is located in the petrous portion of the temporal bone. The inner ear, or labyrinth, is composed of the cochlea, the vestibule, and the semicircular canals (canales semicirculares). The membranous and bony labyrinths contain fluid, called endolymph in the former and perilymph in the latter. Vibrations and currents in this fluid cause stimulation of the sensory cells located in the membranous labyrinth.

Some Figures Concerning the Ear

length of the auricula	6 to 6.5 cm
auditory canal in section	6 to 8 mm
length of the external auditory canal	17 to 24 mm
depth of the middle ear	3 to 6 mm
length of the Eustachian tube	30 to 40 mm
length of the internal auditory canal	4 to 6 mm
length of the cochlea	30 to 35 mm

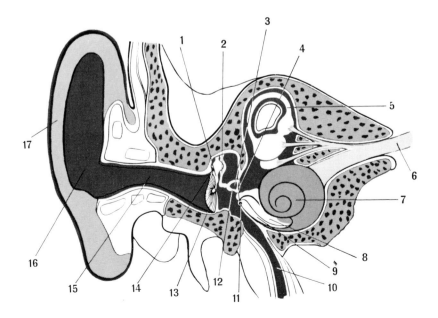

The ear contains two sensory receptor systems: the auditory and the equilibrium organs. The latter is an integral part of the inner auditory organ and both are completely surrounded by bone.

The vestibule of the bony labyrinth is connected posteriorly to the three semicircular canals, each oriented perpendicularly to the other and anteriorly to the coiled cochlea. Between the cochlea and the tympanic cavity is the round window, which is closed by a membrane.

Within the osseous labyrinth two sacs, called the utricle and the saccule, form the membranous labyrinth. From the saccule a duct coiled $2^{1}/_{2}$ times extends anteriorly. In the wall of this coiled duct or cochlea the sensory cells of the auditory organ (organ of Corti) are located. The cochlea consists of a central column around which a bony lamella winds spirally. The membranous cochlea divides the bony cochlea into two parts: an ascending vestibular canal (scala vestibuli) and a descending tympanic cavity canal (scala tympani). At the top of the cochlea the two canals communicate with each other. Vibration transmitted in the fluid of either canal (or scala) can activate the sensory cells of the organ of Corti.

The utricle is located posteriorly in the vestibule and is connected with the three semicircular canals. In the walls of the saccule and utricle and in the three canals the sensory cells of the organ of equilibrium are located. At the point of connection between the canals and the vestibule there is a widening, and in this area cells with long hairs are found. Changes in the position of the head set the fluid in the canals in motion, which causes the hairs to bend. In this way the sensory cells of the organ of equilibrium are stimulated.

The eighth cranial nerve (n. vestibulocochlearis, or vestibulo-cochlear nerve) consists of a vestibular part, which carries the equilibrium stimuli to the brain, and a cochlear part, which carries the stimuli of the auditory organ to the brain.

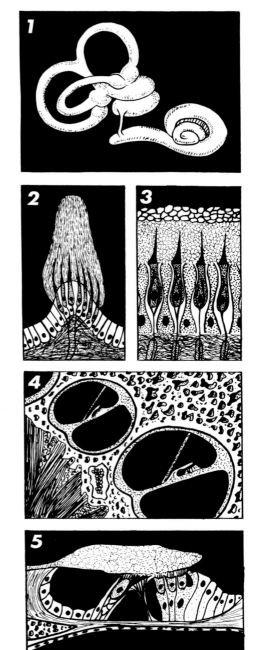

The auditory and equilibrium organs

1. semicircular canals and cochlea
2. and 3. details of the vestibular system
   2: crista
   3: macula
4. and 5. details of the auditory system

←

THE EAR
1. Malleus
   Hammer or malleus
2. Incus
   Anvil or incus
3. M. stapedii
   Stapedius muscle
4. Fenestra ovalis
   Oval window
5. Canalis semicircularis verticalis
   Superior semicircular canal
6. N. vestibulocochlearis
   Vestibulocochlear nerve
7. Cochlea
   Cochlea
8. Scala vestibuli
   Scala vestibuli
9. Scala tympani
   Scala tympani
10. Tuba auditiva
    Auditory or Eustachian tube
11. Fenestra rotunda
    Round window
12. Stapes
    Stirrup or stapes
13. Membrana tympani
    Tympanic membrane
14. M. tensor tympani
    Tensor tympani muscle
15. Meatus acusticus externus
    External auditory meatus
16. Concha auriculae
    Concha of auricula (external ear)
17. Helix auriculae
    Helix of auricula (external ear)

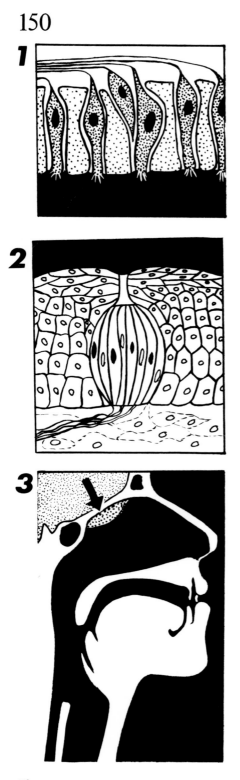

THE NOSE

Man's face is characterized by hairs, a projecting nose and chin, and moving lips. The frontal nasal opening has the shape of an inverted heart. It is bordered by the nasal bones (ossa nasalia) and the upper jaw. The nasal septum is formed by the ethmoid bone and the vomer. Inferiorly, the border of the nasal cavity is formed by two oval openings. The roof consists of the ethmoid bone and the floor is composed of the palatine bone and upper jaw (maxilla). The inner (and largest) section of the nose consists of two cavities, separated by the bony septum. On the outer walls of this area three nasal conchae lie one above the other. The nasal cavity is connected to a number of other cavities or sinuses (frontal, sphenoid, maxillary, and ethmoid).

The three bony folds (conchae) of each nasal cavity are covered by a mucous membrane, in which the olfactory sensory receptors are localized. The olfactory epithelium in man is no larger than 5 cm². The branches of the olfactory nerve (n. olfactorius) arise in this area and the thin, small bundles of nerves perforate the cribriform plate of the ethmoid bone. The stimuli are carried to the central nervous system via the olfactory tract.

Olfactory perception is determined by the receptor cells of the olfactory mucous membrane and the concentration and quality of the substance to be perceived. Our perception of olfactory stimuli is highly developed. Thus, we can perceive 0.000,000,000,002 g of valeric acid in 1 liter of air.

THE TONGUE

The gustatory sensory or taste receptor cells are located primarily in the mucous membrane of the tongue and occasionally in the throat and the palate. On the tongue, four kinds of papillae are found. The mushroom-shaped papillae contain the taste buds with the gustatory sensory cells. They are concentrated on the border of the anterior two-thirds and the posterior end of the tongue. The qualities of taste are distributed over the tongue in a specific manner: sweet at the tip, salty on the edge of the frontal section, and bitter at the back of the tongue. The perception of taste stimuli is supported to a large degree by the sense of smell. The sense of taste tells us nothing about the chemical composition of a substance and is strongly dependent on the concentration; thus 0.02 per cent potassium bromide tastes bittersweet and 0.2 per cent, on the other hand, tastes salty.

The nose

1. olfactory cells
2. gustatory cells
3. nasal cavity (the arrow marks the olfactory epithelium)

PLATE J
EYE
Plaat Nr. 2012

Deutsches Hygiene-Museum,
Dresden

151 – 156

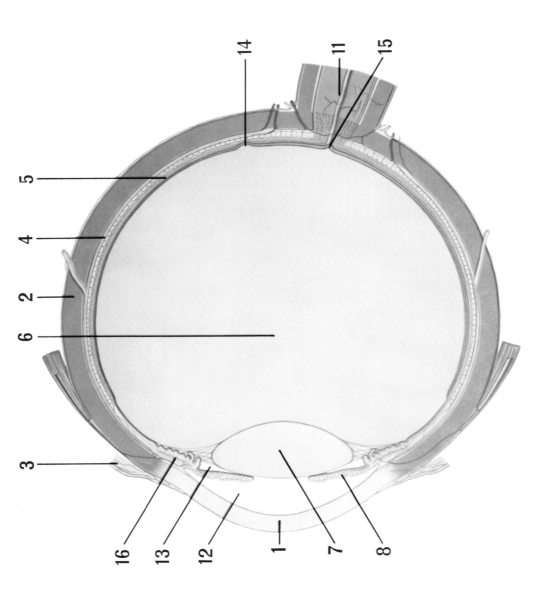

PLATE J
THE EYE

THE EYE

1. Cornea
   Cornea
2. Sclera
   Sclera
3. Tunica conjunctiva
   Ocular conjunctiva
4. Chorioidea
   Chorioid
5. Retina
   Retina
6. Corpus vitreum
   Vitreous body
7. Lens crystallina
   Crystalline lens
8. Iris
   Iris
9. M. sphincter pupillae
   *Pupillary sphincter muscle
   (of iris)*
10. M. ciliaris
    Ciliary muscle
11. N. opticus
    Optic nerve
12. Camera anterior bulbi
    Anterior chamber of the eye
13. Camera posterior bulbi
    Posterior chamber of the eye
14. Fovea centralis
    Fovea centralis of retina
15. Discus n. optici
    Optic disk
16. Corpus ciliare
    Ciliary body
17. M. levator palpebrae superior
    *Levator palpebrae superior
    muscle*
18. Insertio m. obliqui superioris
    *Insertion of superior oblique
    muscle*
19. M. rectus superior
    Superior rectus muscle
20. M. rectus medialis
    Medial rectus muscle
21. M. rectus lateralis
    Lateral rectus muscle
22. M. rectus inferior
    Inferior rectus muscle

The skin of man is a complex organ composed of several layers which cover the exterior body surface: an epithelial layer (epidermis) and a connective tissue layer (dermis), with a subcutaneous connective tissue (subcutis) joining it to the underlying muscle and other tissues.

The skin serves many functions, such as cold, heat and touch reception, temperature regulation, excretion, and protection from damaging substance. The epidermis is divided into two layers — an outer, keratinized layer consisting of flattened cornified cells, and the lower germinal layer consisting of cuboidal and cylindrical cells which are transformed into cornified cells. In the dermis, which indents the epidermis with cone-shaped papillae, blood vessels, nerves, and sensory receptors are localized. The skin is an important sensory organ: touch, pressure, pain, and temperature changes are perceived by receptors located in the skin. Painful stimuli are received through the terminal endings of special sensory nerves, located between the epithelial cells of the epidermis. There are special sensory organs in the dermis of the skin for the reception of other sensory stimuli. The most important of these are:

— Meissner's corpuscles (branching, coiled nerve endings with a connective tussue sheath), respond to touch
— Vater-Pacini's corpuscles (nerve endings which lie encapsulated in a number of concentric shells of connective tissue), respond to pressure
— Krause's corpuscles (nerve branchings surrounded by spherical connective tissue capsule), respond to cold
— Ruffini's corpuscles (richly branching nerve endings surrounded by a connective tissue capsule), respond to heat

The color of the skin is mainly determined by the presence of skin pigment (melanin) and, to a lesser degree, by the blood supply and the thickness of the cornified layer. Also parts of the skin are nails, hair, and glands. The nails consist of cone-shaped, cornified upper skin cells, which are generated in the nail root and lie on the nail bed until forward growth results in a free edge. The toenails are stronger than the fingernails. In an adult, the rate of nail growth is approximately 0.1 mm per day. The hair also is made up of cone-shaped cells. Except for a few places, the whole body is covered by different types of hair: long hair on the head and face, short, stout hair of the eyelids and eyebrows and fine hair covering most of the body. Sebaceous glands, which keep the hair oily, discharge into the hair follicle. Small hair muscles, composed of smooth muscle cells, attach themselves to the hair follicles and can cause the hairs to stand upright and pucker the skin (goose flesh). The many sweat glands (varying from 50 per cm³ on the skin of the back to 400 per cm³ on the inside of the hand) each discharge independently at the surface of the skin.

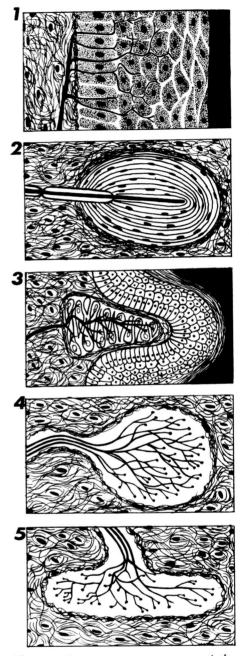

The most important sensory organs of the skin:

1. pain receptor (free nerve-ending)
2. pressure receptor (Vater-Pacini's corpuscle)
3. taste receptor (Meissner's corpuscle)
4. cold receptor (Krause's corpuscle)
5. heat receptor (Ruffini's corpuscle)

A discussion of the senses is inadequate without a review of the cranial nerves, which carry stimuli from the most important sense organs (eye, ear, nose, tongue, and skin) to the brain. Following is a brief review of the twelve cranial nerves, including those which have a motor or secretory function.

First cranial nerve, olfactory nerve (n. olfactorius)

This sensory nerve carries stimuli to the olfactory part of the brain. All nerves carry stimuli in the form of electrical signals. The fibers of this nerve pass from the olfactory mucous membrane, situated in the back of the nose, through the ethmoid bone, where they divide into three branches which go to different areas of the brain. An important olfactory area is situated in the temporal lobe of the cerebrum.

Second cranial nerve, optic nerve (n. opticus)

From the retina, the fibers pass via the optic foramen to the base of the cerebrum. Adjacent to the hypophysis fibers coming from the medial half (on the nasal side) of the retina cross to the opposite side (optic chiasm). The fibers now follow two paths. One leads via a nucleus in the diencephalon (called the lateral geniculate body or *corpus geniculatum laterale*) to the cortex of the occipital lobe in the cerebrum. Every point of the retina is projected onto a specific area of the cerebral cortex. From the other path, some fibers run to the midbrain where they form a component of eye reflexes.

Third cranial nerve, oculomotor nerve (n. oculomotorius)

This motor nerve, together with the fourth and sixth cranial nerves, innervates the six small extrinsic muscles in the eye, which move the eye in all directions. The nuclei for this nerve lie in the midbrain. The oculomotor nerve innervates the superior rectus, inferior rectus, medial rectus, and inferior oblique muscles.

Fourth cranial nerve, trochlear nerve (n. trochlearis)

This is a motor nerve which innervates the superior oblique eye muscle. The tendon of this muscle runs through a circle of connective tissue, which serves as a pulley.

Fifth cranial nerve, trigeminal nerve (n. trigeminus)

This mixed nerve consists of three large sensory branches and a small motor branch. The sensory branches innervate the face, mouth and nasal cavity. The motor nerve innervates the masticatory and several other muscles.

Sixth cranial nerve, abducens nerve (n. abducens)

This motor nerve innervates the lateral rectus eye muscle (m. rectus lateralis), which makes the eye move laterally.

Seventh cranial nerve, facial nerve (n. facialis)

This is a mixed nerve, with a motor part and a sensory part. The nuclei of the motor part lie below the fourth ventricle of the cerebrum. The nerve appears on the lower side of the pons, runs for a short distance in the base of the skull, and gives off many small branches. The facial nerve innervates the facial muscles and a number of glands. The sensory part conducts taste stimuli to the central nervous system.

Eighth cranial nerve, acoustic or vestibulocochlear (n. vestibulocochlearis)

This nerve has two divisions:
a. the cochlear nerve (n. cochlearis), for the sense of hearing
b. the vestibular nerve (n. vestibularis), for registering and transmission of equilibrium stimuli.

The fibers of the auditory nerve end in two nuclei, located in the brain stem. From there, the fibers go either to a reflex center in the midbrain or to a nucleus in the diencephalon (medial geniculate body), after which they go to the auditory area of the temporal lobe. The fibers of the vestibular nerve end in four nuclei in the brain stem, from which they extend into the spinal cord, the cerebellum, and other parts of the brain stem.

Ninth cranial nerve, glossopharyngeal nerve (n. glossopharyngeus)

In certain regards, the ninth and tenth cranial nerves belong together. The nuclei of both nerves are closely associated. Immediately bordering each other, the nerves leave the brain stem and pass through the base of the skull, via the jugular foramen (foramen jugulare). The motor portion partially supplies the pharynx, while other branches innervate the secretory cells of the parotid (salivary) gland and conduct the taste stimuli from the tongue.

Tenth cranial nerve, vagus nerve (n. vagus)

The branches of this important nerve extend to a large area of the body. The vagus innervates the head and neck, and the organs located in the chest and abdomen.

Eleventh cranial nerve, accessory nerve (n. accessorius)

The cells of origin of this nerve are located in the spinal cord as well as in the brain stem. Two muscles, the sternocleidomastoid (m. sternocleidomastoideus) and the trapezius (m. trapezius), are innervated by the accessory nerve.

Twelfth cranial nerve, hypoglossal nerve (n. hypoglossus)

The nucleus of the hypoglossal nerve has an elongated form. This nerve supplies all tongue muscles.

INTERNAL ORGANS

The thoracic and abdominal cavities contain a number of organs, which regulate many essential life functions.

The thoracic cavity contains the organs concerned with respiration and blood circulation, and parts of other systems such as the esophagus. These vulnerable organs are protected by a bony structure, consisting of the ribs, the sternum, and part of the vertebral column. This area is separated from the abdominal cavity by the muscular diaphragm.

The abdominal cavity contains the organs of digestion and excretion. Also present are the liver, gallbladder and spleen, and a number of glands, e.g., the pancreas and the adrenals. In the lowest part of the abdominal cavity (pelvic region) the bladder, a portion of the intestinal system, and an important part of the sexual apparatus are located. The organs of the upper abdomen are partly protected by the ribs, and those in the lower abdomen are protected by the pelvic bones. The greater part of the abdominal cavity is covered by a number of abdominal muscles running in various directions. On the posterior or dorsal side of the body the vertebral column provides a flexible but extremely strong support.

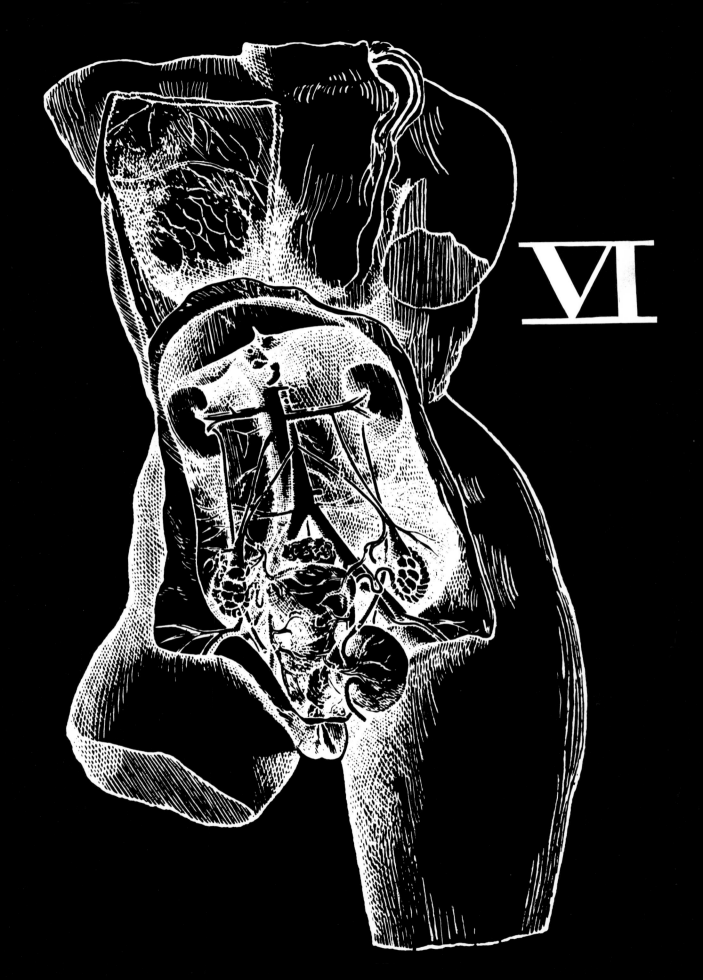

VI

THE TRUNK

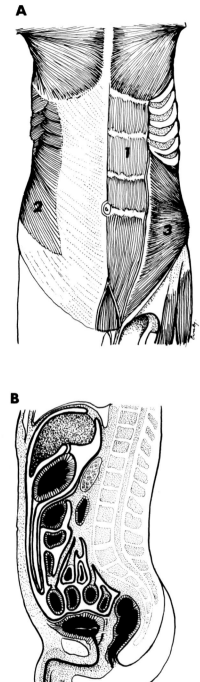

The trunk is the central part of the body and is situated between the shoulder and the pelvis. Topographically, we can distinguish three groups of organs: the chest organs, in the thoracic cavity; the abdominal organs, in the abdominal cavity; and the pelvic organs, in the pelvic cavity. The skeleton of the trunk is formed by part of the vertebral column, the ribs, and the sternum.

The upper part of the trunk, the chest or thorax, consists of a bony thorax, outside of which the many chest muscles are found. The most important organs belonging to the thoracic cavity are the heart and the lungs. In the area between the lungs but containing the heart (mediastinum) large veins and arteries, the windpipe (trachea) and the esophagus are found. This area is separated from the abdominal cavity by the diaphragm, a large flat muscle which not only fulfills an important task in regard to controlling respiration, but also plays a role in determining intra-abdominal pressure. In the diaphragm we find a number of openings for large vessels, nerves and the esophagus.

The abdomen is not completely surrounded by bony structures but has a bony support on its posterior side. Furthermore, the abdominal wall is composed of a number of muscles with fibers extending in several directions. Just as in the thoracic cavity, the inner surface of the abdomen is also lined by a membrane, which in this case is called the peritoneum. The abdominal cavity contains, in the upper right quadrant, the liver and gallbladder; in the upper left quadrant, the stomach; in the upper left "posterior" quadrant, the spleen, adrenal glands, and kidneys; and below, ventrally in the midline, the bladder. The remaining area is filled by the intestines, while the internal sexual organs are found in the pelvis.

The ventral portion of the abdominal wall is the rectus abdominus muscle (m. rectus abdominis), running to the right and to the left of the midline and attached to the cartilage of the lower ribs and sternum and below to the upper edge of the pubic bone (os pubis). Next to this muscle lie three broad abdominal muscles:

a. external oblique abdominal muscle (m. obliquus externus abdominis), which runs from the ribs to the wall of the iliac bone (os ilium); the direction of the fibers is from upper-lateral to lower-medial;
b. internal oblique abdominal muscle (m. obliquus internus abdominis), which runs from the medial side or costal cartilage of the three lower ribs to the ilium and some nearby structures;
c. transverse abdominal muscle (m. transversus abdominis), which arises, along with others, on the ilium and the ribs, and crosses medially into the sheath surrounding the rectus abdominus muscle.

The most important muscle of the posterior part of the abdominal wall is the quadrilateral lumbar muscle (m. quadratus lumborum), which extends from the interior border of the lower rib to the transverse processes of the lower three lumbar vertebrae and the crest of the ilium.

The muscles form a flexible enclosure for the abdominal cavity to accommodate the changing content of the abdominal organs, to permit bending of the trunk, and to support the vertebral column.

A. *Abdominal muscles*
1. rectus abdominis muscle
2. external oblique muscle
3. internal oblique muscle
B. *Median section through the abdominal cavity*
The organs seen in section are surrounded by the peritoneum.

The organ system involved in the digestion of food consists of a specialized canal (alimentary canal) which begins in the oral cavity and ends at the anal opening (anus). A large number of organs form this system and they fulfill a series of functions: ingestion of food, mechanical processing and chemical digestion, transport of digested food through the intestinal walls for absorption in the blood and lymphatic vessels, and expulsion of the undigested residue. Other organs are connected by ducts with the digestive tract; the substances produced by these organs aid the digestive process.

Functionally, the whole system is made up of three parts: in the upper section (oral cavity and pharynx, stomach and duodenum), the mechanical and chemical processing of the food components takes place; in the middle section (the small intestine), the transportation of the small, digested food particles through the intestinal wall takes place; and in the last section (large intestine, rectum and anus), the indigestible remainder is stored, transported and expelled from the body. A dehydration process, in which much water is withdrawn for the contents of the large intestine, also takes place.

On its way from the oral cavity to the anus, the food passes the following components of the digestive tract:

— oral cavity with tongue and palate, teeth and salivary glands;
— esophagus;
— stomach;
— small intestine:
    duodenum, into which discharge the excretory ducts of the liver (gallbladder) and the pancreatic gland,
    jejunum,
    ileum;
— large intestine:
    cecum,
    appendix,
    ascending colon (colon ascendens),
    transverse colon (colon transversum),
    descending colon (colon descendens),
    sigmoid colon (colon sigmoideum);
— rectum and anal opening (anus).

The many glands associated with the digestive tract generally produce enzymes which exert a catalytic effect upon one of the phases of the digestive process of the most important food components such as carbohydrates, fats and proteins. Scientists still use the old-fashioned word "juice" to describe the fluid containing a complex mixture of salts and protein enzymes; thus, the glands of the stomach wall are said to produce gastric juice, the pancreatic gland produces pancreatic juice, and the glands of the intestinal wall produce intestinal juice.

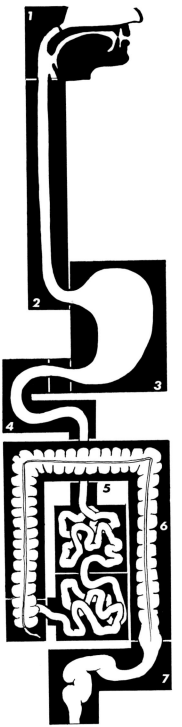

Schematic representation of the digestive tract

1. oral cavity and pharynx
2. esophagus
3. stomach
4. duodenum
5. small intestine
6. large intestine
7. rectum

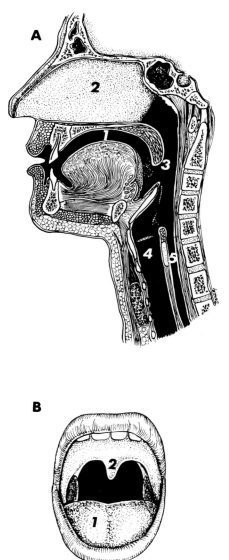

In the oral cavity the food is finely ground, with the help of the teeth and tongue, and mixed with saliva. The tongue is composed of intrinsic muscles and extrinsic muscles, which allow it great mobility. This organ, covered by mucous membrane, serves for sucking, chewing and swallowing of food, and for speech. The oral cavity is bordered on both sides by two palatal arches. Between the arches lie the palatine tonsils *(tonsillae palatinae)*. The *pharynx* is the area posterior or dorsal to the oral and nasal cavities; below, it extends into the *esophagus* and, via the larynx, into the windpipe *(trachea)*. Food passage (oral cavity — esophagus and air passage (nasal cavity — larynx) are separated from each other in this area. The food is brought to the esophagus by the tongue and the muscles in the wall of the pharynx; swallowing is a reflex action.

The esophagus, with a length of approximately 25 cm and a width of approximately 2 cm, has a strong, smooth muscle wall which transports food to the stomach by means of peristaltic movements.

Directly under the diaphragm, the esophagus has an outlet into the cardia antrum (entrance) of the stomach. Here the food is mixed with gastric juice containing hydrochloric acid and enzymes. The stomach wall, made up of three layers of muscles, contracts forcefully, and the food passes through the relaxed pylorus into the duodenum. The mucous membrane of the empty stomach is prominently folded. The exit of the stomach, the *pylorus,* consists of a strong sphincter muscle which relaxes for short periods of time in order to let pass small portions of chyme.

The first section of the small intestine is the *duodenum,* an arched tube in the shape of a horseshoe, located behind the peritoneum and joined by connective tissue to the posterior wall of the abdomen, and into which the ducts of the liver and the pancreatic gland discharge their products (bile and digestive enzymes respectively).

The small intestine has a length of four to five meters, and, in order to have the greatest possible surface for the transport of digested food through the intestinal wall, it is strongly convoluted and provided with a large number of folds (Kerckring's folds). From the surface, countless villi increase the surface area to facilitate the absorption of digested food. The smooth muscles serve in mixing the chyme as well as in its transport by means of peristaltic movements. This double muscle function is brought about by a layer of longitudinal and circular smooth muscles. The intestinal wall further shows a large number of tubular sacs (Lieberkühn's crypts), in which the intestinal juices are excreted. The intestinal wall is innervated by the autonomic nervous system, which forms many plexuses between the different layers of the wall.

A. *Transverse section through the head*

1. oral cavity
2. nasal cavity
3. pharynx
4. trachea
5. esophagus

B. *View inside the mouth*
1. tongue
2. uvula

PLATE K
INTERNAL ORGANS OF MAN

Plaat Nr. 2006
Deutsches Hygiene-Museum,
Dresden

165–170

P L A T E K
INTERNAL ORGANS OF MAN

1. Ventriculus sinister
   Left ventricle
2. Ventriculus dexter
   Right ventricle
3. Apex cordis
   Apex of the heart
4. Mm. papillares
   Papillary muscles
5. Septum interventriculare
   Ventricular septum
6. Valvula atrioventricularis dextra
   Tricuspid valve
7. Valvula atrioventricularis sinistra
   Bicuspid valve (mitral)
8. Atrium dextrum
   Right atrium
9. Atrium sinistrum
   Left atrium
10. Pericardium
    Pericardium

11. Vv. pulmonales
    Pulmonary veins
12. Aorta ascendens
    Ascending aorta
13. A. pulmonalis
    Pulmonary artery
14. V. cava superior
    Superior vena cava
15. Arcus aortae
    Aortic arch
16. Truncus brachiocephalicus
    Innominate artery
17. A. carotis communis
    Common carotid artery
18. A. subclavia sinistra
    Left subclavian artery
19. A. carotis communis dextra
    Right common carotid artery
20. A. carotis communis sinistra
    Left common carotid artery

21. A. subclavia dextra
    Right subclavian artery
22. V. jugularis interna
    Internal jugular vein
23. V. subclavia dextra
    Right subclavian vein
24. V. subclavia sinistra
    Left subclavian vein
25. Trachea
    Trachea
26. V. jugularis externa
    External jugular vein
27. Larynx
    Larynx
28. Clavicula
    Collarbone
29. Apex pulmonis
    Apex of lung
30. Bronchus principalis (dexter)
    Right bronchus
31. Pulmo dexter
    Right lung
32. Pulmo sinister
    Left lung
33. Diaphragma
    Diaphragm
34. Hepar
    Liver
35. Vv. hepatica
    Hepatic veins
36. V. portae
    Portal vein

37. A. hepatica propria
    Hepatic artery
38. Vesica fellea
    Gallbladder
39. Ductus choledochus
    Common bile duct
40. Ventriculus (gaster)
    Stomach
41. Lien
    Spleen
42. A. lienalis
    Splenic artery
43. V. lienalis
    Splenic vein
44. Duodenum
    Duodenum
45. Pancreas
    Pancreas
46. Ductus pancreaticus
    Pancreatic duct
47. Ren
    Kidney
48. Mesocolon
    Mesocolon
49. Ileum
    Ileum
50. Caecum
    Cecum
51. Appendix vermiformis
    Vermiform appendix
52. Taenia coli
    Tenia coli

53. Colon ascendens
    Ascending colon
54. Colon transversum
    Transverse colon
55. Colon descendens
    Descending colon
56. Colon sigmoideum
    Sigmoid colon
57. Rectum
    Rectum
58. Ureter
    Ureter
59. Vesica urinaria
    Urinary bladder
60. Aorta abdominalis
    Abdominal aorta
61. A. mesenterica inferior
    Inferior mesenteric artery
62. A. testicularis
    Internal spermatic artery
63. A. iliaca communis
    Common iliac artery
64. A. iliaca externa
    External iliac artery
65. V. cava inferior
    Inferior vena cava
66. V. iliaca communis
    Common iliac vein
67. V. iliaca externa
    External iliac vein
68. V. testicularis dextra
    Spermatic vein

The excretory duct of the gallbladder *(ductus choledochus)* and that of the pancreas *(ductus pancreaticus)* discharge jointly into the duodenum, in a place which is marked by a small elevation, *Vater's papilla.*

The liver *(hepar),* which is the largest gland of the body (approximately 1½ kg), lies above the abdomen to the right, directly below the diaphragm. This organ is made up of a number of lobes which are further divided into countless liver lobules and units, held together by connective tissue. Each such unit is spanned by a network of capillaries, coming from the portal vein (which transports the digested food) and the hepatic artery (the liver artery which transports oxygen-rich blood).

Between the liver cells lie the bile capillaries which unite as bile ducts, and eventually leave the liver as a common hepatic duct *(ductus hepaticus).* A side arm of this duct, the cystic duct *(ductus cysticus),* is joined to the gallbladder *(vesica fellae).* This pear-shaped organ, which stores bile, has a volume of about 35 cc. The liver continually produces bile, but the gallbladder discharges bile into the duodenum only after a meal; this is assisted by muscle contractions of the gallbladder wall. The *pancreas* is an oblong organ, located in the curve of the duodenum, posteriorly behind the peritoneum. This gland releases the pancreatic juice via the pancreatic duct; the enzyme-rich juice is important for the breakdown of proteins, fats and carbohydrates. Two hormones, insulin and glucagon, are also pancreatic products and both are delivered into the blood stream. They play an important role in the metabolism of carbohydrates.

The small intestine passes into the large instestine in such a way that a blind pouch *(cecum)* is formed in the large intestine. The vermiform (worm-shaped) *appendix* is another blind pouch that is joined to the cecum. In the large intestine, the chyme comes into contact with bacteria which, among other things, can break down cellulose, a component of plant cells (vegetables). The passage between the small and large intestines contains a valve (ileocecal valve) which prevents the contents of the colon from passing backward into the ileum, the distal end of the small intestine. The surface of the large intestine *(colon)* has many ridges and constrictions but it has no villi. There are several segments to be distinguished in the colon: on the right side in the abdominal cavity is the ascending colon *(colon ascendens),* then a segment which runs from upper right to upper left *(colon transversum),* and finally a descending segment *(colon descendens)* on the left side. The terminal section is an S-shaped curve *(colon sigmoideum)* and continues into the *rectum.* The rectum lies against the posterior wall of the pelvis, bends posteriorly and ends as the *anus.* The circular muscle layer of the colon is thickened at the anus to form a sphincter muscle *(sphincter internus).* A striated muscle *(sphincer externus),* which forms part of the floor of the pelvis, is under voluntary control and regulates the opening and closing of the anal orifice.

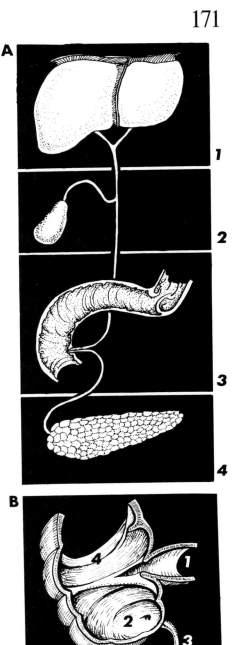

A. *Section of the digestive system*
1. the liver and its excretory ducts
2. the gallbladder
3. the duodenum with the excretory ducts of the liver and pancreas
4. the pancreas and its excretory duct to the duodenum

B. *The transition from small to large intestine*
1. terminal section of the small intestine (ileum)
2. cecum in blind pouch
3. vermiform appendix
4. large intestine

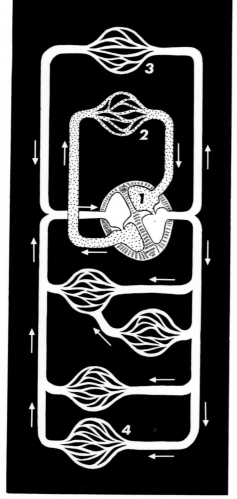

Schema of the large and small circulation systems

1. the heart
2. pulmonary circulation system
3. vascular bed of the head
4. vascular bed of the trunk and extremities

On pages 000, 000, 000 most of the important blood vessels of the human body can be found. The blood is kept in movement by contraction of the heart muscle, and by valves in the heart which allow the blood to flow in only one direction. The heart, an organ the size of a human fist, consists of two synchronously working doubleacting pumps, lying next to each other.

The heart viewed frontally has the shape of a tilted three-sided cone. It lies on the diaphragm with its tip or apex directed toward the left, away from the midline. The movement of the heart during contraction (the beating of the heart against the wall of the chest) can be felt in the fifth intercostal area, to the left, below the nipple. The base of the heart is located at the level of the third rib, posteriorly and laterally to the right. From this base the great veins (inflow) and arteries (outflow) enter and leave the heart. The heart is protected by the ribs and sternum (breastbone); it reaches from the second intercostal space to the lower side of the fifth rib and is partly located behind the breastbone and the left ribs.

Four chambers can be distinguished in the heart: left *atrium* and *ventricle,* and right atrium and ventricle. The right and left halves of the heart are separated from each other by a septum. The two chambers of the left heart are separated by the bicuspid valve or mitral valve *(valva mitralis);* and between the chambers of the right heart is found the tricuspid valve *(valva tricuspidalis).* Also between the two ventricles and the arteries, valves are found which prevent the backflow of blood after contraction empties the chambers. Between the right ventricle and the pulmonary artery, and between the left ventricle and the aorta, are valves of analogous structure, the semilunar valves *(valvulae semilunares),* formed in the shape of half-moons.

The blood of the systemic venous system, poor in oxygen, is gathered in both caval veins *(v. cava superior* and *v. cava inferior)* and fills the right atrium with a continuous flow. The oxygen-rich blood from the lungs streams into the left atrium via the pulmonary veins. In this manner, the heart is connected in two places (body and pulmonary systems) to the circular course of the blood; the path is as follows: venous blood vessels — right half of the heart — lung vessels — left half of the heart — arterial body vessels — capillaries — and back into the venous system for recirculation.

The heart is built up of three layers: an inner wall and valves *(endocardium),* muscle layer *(myocardium),* and the pericardial sac *(pericardium).* The wall of the left heart is significantly thicker than that of the right heart. The muscle layer is thickest in the left ventricle and thin in both atria.

The heart muscle itself receives blood through the right and left coronary arteries *(a. coronaria),* which arise from the aorta directly above the semilunar valves.

This organ system supplies oxygen to and removes carbon dioxide from the blood. The air we breathe is a mixture of oxygen, carbon dioxide, nitrogen, and inert gases in variable percentages. The respiratory system can be divided into two groups of organs: *upper air passages,* including the nasal cavity and pharynx, larynx and trachea; and the *lower air passages,* including the bronchi, bronchioles, and alveoli.

NASAL CAVITY - PHARYNX

The nasal cavity is divided by a septum into a left and a right half. The mucous membrane of the frontal section of the cavity is covered by ciliated and mucus-producing cells. On the side walls are found three *conchae,* which narrow the nasal cavity. The mucous membrane of the nasal cavity has a very rich blood supply: under the middle and upper conchae the outlets of other cavities (sinuses) serve to warm inhaled air, while under the lowest concha is located the outlet of the lacrimal canal, through which tear fluid from the eye is conducted into the nasal cavity to be evaporated, on inhalation of dry air, in order to elevate the humidity. Through these structures, the inhaled air is brought to the right levels of temperature and moisture, and is also cleaned of dust and bacteria.

The pharynx is an area surrounded by striated muscle, and has in its wall a number of tonsillar masses (tonsillae), accumulations of lymphatic tissue, which destroy bacteria.

LARYNX

The larynx connects the pharynx to the trachea, or windpipe. It is here that the vocal cords are found and where speech is made possible. The whole organ is made up of a number of bones, cartilages, and muscles, which are connected to each other in a complicated manner and which can be moved with respect to each other. The thyroid cartilage *(cartilago thyroidea)* and below it the ring-shaped cartilage *(cartilago cricoidea)* are the most important.

The entrance to the larynx is closed by the *epiglottis,* which moves upward when swallowing takes place, closing off this area, so that no food can enter the windpipe. Between the thyroid cartilage and the cup-shaped cartilage, the vocal cords are stretched and can vibrate when air is expired. The cords run in an anterior-posterior direction and between them a narrow opening, the glottis rima glottidis, is located. The opening can be narrowed and widened by muscular contraction or relaxation. Chest, lips, tongue and palate also play important roles in sound (voice) production.

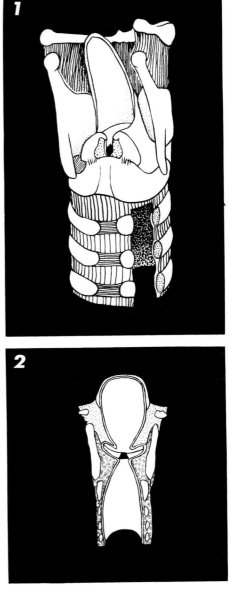

The larynx, which forms the connection between the pharynx and the windpipe

1. frontal and side view
2. section

TRACHEA AND LUNGS

The windpipe *(trachea),* a duct 12 cm long, is strengthened by 18 to 20 incomplete cartilaginous rings joined together by mouth muscle and strong elastic connective tissue. At the level of the fifth thoracic vertebra the trachea divides (bifurcates) into two main bronchi which penetrate the left and right lungs at the lung hilus. The lung hilus is also the point of entrance and exit of the arteries and veins of the lungs. The main bronchus branches in the lung like a tree; the left main bronchus splits into two branches and the right into three, forming the major lung segments. These bronchi possess complete cartilaginous rings and a layer of smooth muscle, and are lined internally with cylindrical epithelial cells which remove dust particles from the inhaled air in the lungs with cilia covering their free surface.

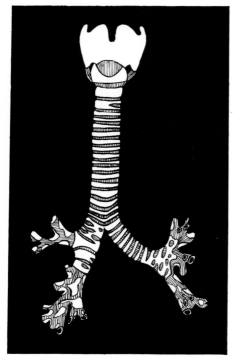

A. *The trachea with its most important branches*

BRONCHI

The bronchi pass into the bronchioles, which become increasingly narrow and eventually end in thin-walled vesicles *(alveoli).* In total, there are between 500,000,000 and 600,000,000 alveoli which have a total surface of 130 to 150 m². The alveoli are surrounded by a network of capillaries which is very efficient for the exchange of oxygen and carbon dioxide.

LUNGS

The lungs and the heart occupy the major part of the thoracic cavity. The remaining area is filled with nerves and blood vessels. The right lung consists of three lobes: an upper, middle and lower; and the left lung of two lobes: an upper and a lower. The lungs are completely surrounded by a flattened sac or membrane *(pleura),* the walls of which are designated as the parietal pleura *(pleura parietalis),* the outer wall lining the inner surface of the thoracic cavity and the visceral pleura *(pleura visceralis),* the inner wall adhering directly to the lung.

The thoracic cavity and associated muscles are as important as the lungs for respiration: inspiration results from muscular activity, while expiration is passive and due mainly to the elasticity of the lungs.

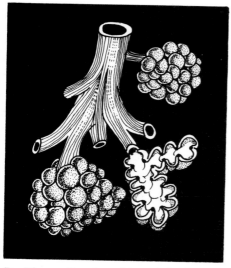

B. *The smallest branching of the bronchioles, which continue into the alveoli*

The kidneys, ureters, bladder, and urethra form the excretory apparatus of man. The most important task of the apparatus is that of purifying the blood and eliminating waste products.

Both kidneys *(renes),* located at the posterior side of the abdominal cavity, are bean-shaped organs reaching from the eleventh or twelfth rib to the third lumbar vertebra. The left kidney lies somewhat higher than the right kidney. Its medial side has a cavity from which the *ureter* and the renal vein *(v. renalis)* exit and the renal artery *(a. renalis)* enters the kidney.

In cross section, the kidney is seen to possess a cortex and a medulla. In the cortex lie over 1 million glomeruli, containing finely branching capillary plexuses which come in close contact with the cup-shaped, double-walled sac (Bowman's capsule) of the *nephron* which serves the complicated filtration and reabsorption processes of the kidney. In the *medulla,* parallel-arranged excretory ducts are situated, all of which open from a central gathering point: the kidney and pelvis. Here is gathered the urine which flows via the ureter to the bladder.

The *ureters* are hollow ducts, 25 to 35 cm in length, which arise in the kidney and pelvis, run beside the vertebral column along the posterior abdominal wall, and then take an oblique direction along the lateral wall of the pelvis to enter the posterior surface of the wall of the bladder. Several layers of smooth muscle fibers in the wall of the ureter move the urine to the bladder by peristalsis.

The bladder *(vesica urinaria)* is a hollow organ, situated behind the pubic symphyses. The wall is formed of three layers of smooth muscle fibers which enable this organ to adapt easily to a changing volume. The urine drips continuously into the bladder and, when it is filled to approximately 400 cc, nerves are stimulated and the bladder contraction is set into motion. At the junction of the bladder with the urethra, a muscular sphincter is situated; this muscle prevents the urine from flowing out of the bladder. The capacity of the bladder, depending on age, is 200 to 900 cc. An empty bladder is an organ the size of an orange with a very thick wall.

The *urethra* is shorter in the woman than in the man. The female urethra follows a straight course and discharges from the vaginal vestibule. The male urethra has a double bend and serves not only in the transportation of urine but also of sperm. The urethra perforates the floor of the pelvis, a complex of membranes and muscles which close off the pelvic exit.

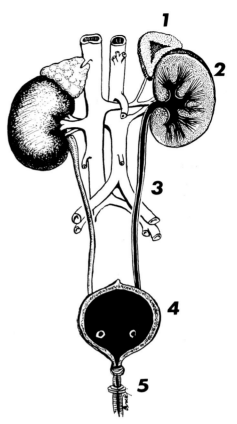

Schematic drawing of the excretory organs

1. suprarenal gland (an essential endocrine gland but does not belong to the urinary apparatus)
2. kidney
3. ureter
4. bladder
5. urethra

GENITAL ORGANS

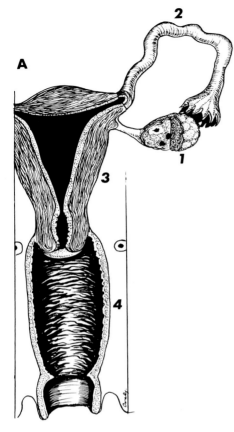

The female sex organs consist of the *internal organs* (ovaries, oviducts, uterus, and vagina) and the *external organs* (labia, clitoris, and mons pubis). The sexual glands (ovaries or *ovaria*) are small, almond-shaped organs, situated against the lateral wall of the pelvis, and attached by cords and folds of the peritoneum. The contents of the ovaries, with the exception of connective tissue, blood vessels, etc., consist of ova of differing sizes, representing different stages of development. The more mature ova lie nearer to the ovarian surface, surrounded by supporting follicular cells. In a sexually mature woman, such a follicle ruptures and an ovum is discharged approximately every four weeks *(ovulation)*. After discharge the ovum is carried along by the cilia of the oviduct. The time of ovulation lies approximately midway between two menstruations. The oviduct (Fallopian tube, *tuba uterina),* 10 to 20 cm long, conducts the ovum to the uterus. The beginning of the oviduct is widened into the shape of a trumpet, and is provided with small processes (fimbriae) which facilitate passage of the ovum. Fertilization generally takes place in the oviduct, after which the ovum becomes imbedded in the wall of the uterus.

The fertilized ovum reaches full development in the womb *(uterus).* The uterus is a pear-shaped organ, 8 to 10 cm long, with a thick wall (relaxed, 1 to 2 mm) and a cavity in the form of a triangular cleft. It is situated in the middle of the pelvis and is attached to its lateral walls by means of a fold of the peritoneum. If a fertilized cell develops fully, the wall of the uterus is very much stretched and contractions of the muscle wall (birth pains) force the expulsion of the child through the vagina. If fertilization has not taken place, the ovum degenerates and is eliminated from the uterus, together with some mucous membrane from the uterus during *menstruation* (monthly bleeding).

The narrow, lower section of the uterus, the *cervix* (= neck), protrudes into the vagina. The *vagina* is a duct (10 to 13 cm long), lined with mucous membrane and a muscular wall. At the lower end of the vagina is an outlet into the vaginal vestibule *(portio)* which, in young girls, is usually partially closed off by a membrane *(hymen).*

The vaginal vestibule is surrounded on both sides by a skin fold *(labia minora).* These folds come together anteriorly, at a point, where a small erectile organ *(clitoris)* is located. Beneath the clitoris lies the urethral orifice.

The *labia majora* border the pubic cleft and also, to a large degree, lie across the labia minora and the clitoris. In a sexually mature woman the *mons pubis* and the labia majora are covered with hair.

The female sexual organs

A. Frontal section
1. ovary
2. oviduct
3. uterus
4. vagina

B. Transverse section
1. ovary
2. uterus
3. vagina
4. bladder
5. rectum and anal opening

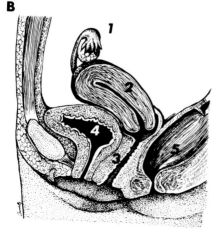

The male sexual organs consist of a sperm-generating and a sperm-discharging portion. The *semen* or sperm is produced in the *testes*, two egg-shaped organs which, surrounded by membranes, are situated externally in the *scrotum*. Both male sex cells and male hormones are produced in the testes. The testis is composed of a number of lobes comprised of many tubules which unite to form a large convoluted discharging duct. This duct *(epididymis)* lies against the testis and contains mature spermatozoa. The testes lie outside the abdominal cavity, because the temperature within the abdomen is too high for the generation, production, and discharge of spermatozoa.

Seminal Duct

The semen in the system of ducts can be discharged by forceful contractions of the *vas deferens*. This duct leaves the scrotum and runs anteriorly along the upper edge of the pubic bone, to reach the abdominal cavity via the inguinal canal. Lateral to the bladder, the seminal ducts curve posteriorly and open into the posterior wall of the urethra. The seminal vesicles *(vesiculae seminales)*, where seminal fluid is produced which promotes the mobility of the spermatozoa, join the vas deferens near its urethral opening.

Prostate

The prostate gland is located at the junction of the vas deferens and the urethra and delivers its secretion into the urethra via a number of small openings.

Penis

The external sexual organ of the human male is the *penis.* It contains three columns of spongy tissue *(corpora cavernosa)*, rich in blood vessels and sinuses which, through certain stimuli, become filled with blood so that a stiffening *(erection)* of the penis occurs. The two upper columns can become very hard, while the lower, in which the urethra runs, and which ends in the *glans,* is less rigid. The glans is surrounded by a skin fold, or prepuce *(preputium)*, which slides back with the swelling of the penis.

The penis has a double function: the transportation of the urine and the transfer of spermatozoa in copulation. The quantity of semen at one ejaculation is approximately 2 to 4 cc, which may contain 400 to 500 million sperm cells.

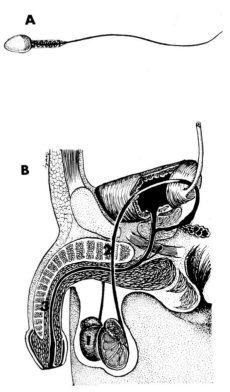

A. *Male sperm cell*

B. *Median section through the male sexual apparatus*

1. testis and epididymis
2. vas deferens
3. penis

178
INDEX

NOTE: This index provides not only the page numbers on which pertinent da can be found but also a key to the four color foldout plates throughout the book. Each capital letter and its following number refer to a specific plate and an item on the plate; e.g., G a 16 following the entry a. angularis denotes that this artery appears on Plate G, and is number 16 in the list of arteries on the plate.

180

182

188